THE
FEELGOOD
PLAN

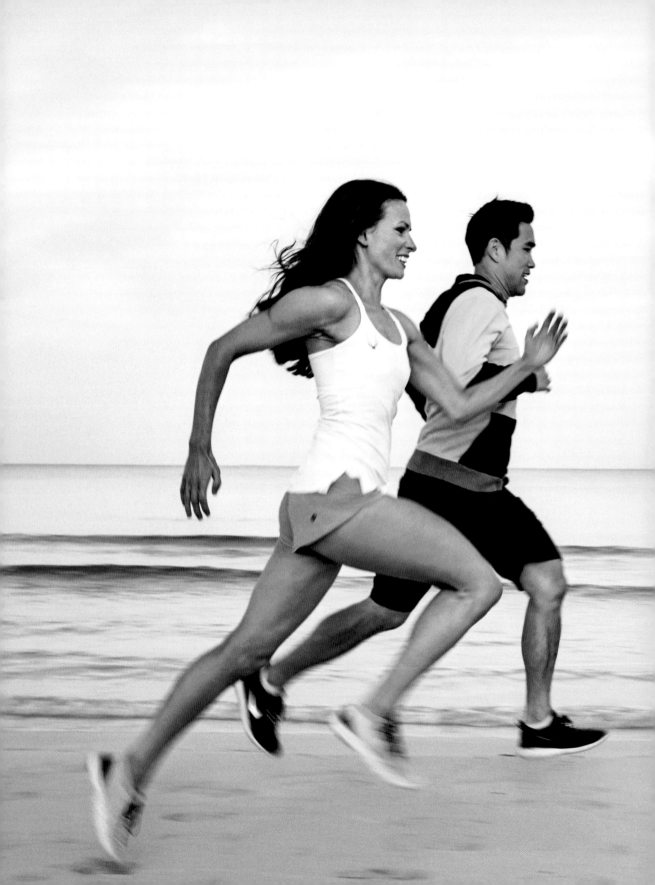

THE FEELGOOD PLAN

Dalton Wong
& Kate Faithfull-Williams

HAPPIER, HEALTHIER & SLIMMER IN

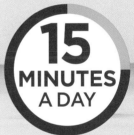

15 MINUTES A DAY

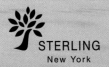

STERLING
New York

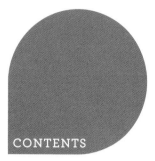

CONTENTS

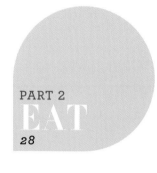

PART 2
EAT
28

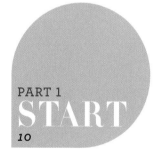

PART 1
START
10

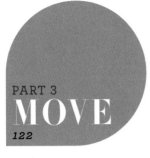

PART 3
MOVE
122

PART 4
RELAX
162

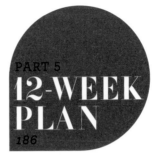

PART 5
12-WEEK PLAN
186

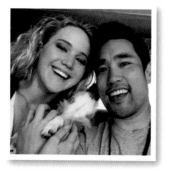

FOREWORD

I met Dalton back in 2010 when he trained me for *X-Men: First Class*. We spent 10–12 hours a day together for three months, working out between filming on set. He changed my body for that movie but gave me the skills to change my life. We remain good friends; when I'm in London I love to train in his gym, then afterwards we go out for burgers and fries with his family. It's all about balance.

Dalton is different to other trainers because he understands what my body needs—how to exercise, when to unwind, how to enjoy food. I could never live on a "diet". Dalton taught me how to eat, move and live a delicious but healthy life. I will always thank him for that.

When we met up on the set of *X-Men: Apocalypse* last summer, we got a chance to catch up. Sometimes hanging out with old friends is more important than exercise. I'm so happy Dalton has written a book with such a wonderful message.

Jennifer Lawrence

MEET THE FEELGOOD PLAN
This book will make you feel good

The feelgood philosophy is simple: when you feel good about yourself, you look your best. This book shows you practical, positive ways to maximize that feelgood sensation and feel a little bit happier and healthier every day.

Sure, weight loss can be one side-effect of living a healthy, happy life, but it's not a goal that overshadows all the fun things. *The Feelgood Plan* is about enjoying life—and your food. This book is not about starvation, polystyrene-flavored rice cakes or unrealistic promises of losing 14lb in 14 days. It's not about a hardcore exercise regime that's actually a one-way ticket to burnout. *The Feelgood Plan* is about taking care of yourself and understanding what your body needs to feel your best.

So if you want to feel happy with your body, try *The Feelgood Plan*. If you love pizza, you'll discover how you can eat it and still be healthy. If you feel powerless in the company of chocolate, you'll develop willpower and learn how to relax around food. If you hate exercise, you'll find the workout that tones you, rather than tortures. If you're too busy (who isn't?) then you'll discover how fitness and nutrition enhance your life, not get in the way of it.

How does it work? By taking 15 minutes—that's just 1% of your day—to do something for your body that makes you feel good. You don't just get an instant lift, you build a lasting change. This book is packed with smart ways to help you tune into what really makes your body happy, from the workout that makes you look and feel younger, to healthy dinners that help you sleep. By making small daily changes to how you eat, exercise and unwind, you'll discover exactly what makes you feel good. The more you do it, the more you'll want to keep doing it. Whenever you feel tired or stressed out, just take 15 minutes to turn your mood around and climb back up towards the feelgood zone.

In Eat, you get makeovers that tweak all your favorite foods so they're better for your body. In Move, you'll find energising and effective exercise plans that are easy to fit into even the most hectic of lives.
In Relax, you learn the secret to enjoying a healthy, happy life beyond

work. At the end you'll find a 12-week plan to put your healthy intentions into action.

When you give your body the nutrition, exercise, rest and compassion it needs to feel good, everything in your whole life becomes easier. Instead of obsessing over January detoxes and summer bikini blitzes, you'll have a slim, strong, healthy body you're happy with all year round. You'll be more productive at work, more relaxed in your relationships, and happier in yourself. And you can still enjoy the foods you love without worrying about your weight.

THE FEELGOOD PLAN DELIVERS ON ITS PROMISE

And these results will last forever. Every tip you read in this book is backed up by sound science and academic studies you can trust. *The Feelgood Plan* is the very opposite of an extreme, quick-fix fad: it is healthy, do-able and sustainable. It's a plan for life.

HOW TO USE THIS BOOK

You don't have to plod through from cover to cover. It will help to read the first two chapters, which lay out the Feelgood philosophy and explain how to get started. From there, if you want to know about, say, controlling cravings, it's OK to turn straight to that chapter. That way, even if you read this book in chunks, you'll understand the ideas in the context of knowing what makes your body feel good—which is how you'll make it happen.

Nature is on your side:
your body is surprisingly well-tuned
to be healthy when you treat it well.

HELLO FROM THE AUTHORS

Dalton Wong is one of the world's leading personal trainers and the founder of Twenty Two Training, a boutique gym in Kensington, London. He has trained royalty, politicians, business leaders and the Hollywood elite.

"My daughter Indigo inspired *The Feelgood Plan*. Aged ten, she recently came home from school upset because another girl had called her fat. I was shocked. But then I put myself in Indigo's tiny shoes and looked around: her view of "normal" is warped. The characters she and her schoolfriends love on TV are unrealistically thin, and those characters talk about their appearance all the time, while the adverts in those same TV shows are for junk food that is scientifically engineered to make you eat more and more of it.

"'You're fat,' is the ultimate insult in a child's world. Right now, the f-word is just that, a word, for Indigo. But chances are that as she grows up she will become more body-conscious. I worry that this could lead to all sorts of psychological and health issues—conditions that can be crippling, yet are worryingly normal for young women.

"So I want to give Indigo the tools to look after her body. I want her to enjoy ice cream as much as she enjoys running around in the park afterwards. I want her to know that wellbeing beats weight, every time. I want everyone to know that having a healthy body is something worth working for, and to be treasured."

Kate Faithfull-Williams is an experienced health and lifestyle journalist. Previously Health Editor of *Grazia* magazine, her work has also been published in *Sunday Times STYLE*, *The Observer*, *The Daily Mail*, *GLAMOUR*, *Cosmopolitan*, *Stylist*, *Fabulous*, *Now*, *Look*, *OK!*, *Top Santé* and *Men's Health*.

"Right up until two weeks before the shoot, Dalton and I assumed we'd have models to do the pictures for our book, but the moment we agreed to have our faces (and thighs and tummies) photographed, it made sense. We're real people, with real bodies. We're living proof that you can find peace with your body, fit exercise into your week, enjoy the foods you love—and have a life.

"Before getting married in 2011, I met Dalton through my work as a health editor and I asked him to shave off the stubborn 5 lbs standing in the way of me and my dream wedding dress. Instead of treating me like a number on the scales, Dalton figured out my weight wasn't the real issue. I was bloated, tired and suffered nagging back pain. I was uptight about what my weight "should" be. I was also inclined to eat giant bowls of cereal late at night if anyone told me carbs were off-limits. If I knew a colleague had chocolate stashed in her drawer, I couldn't concentrate on my job.

"Dalton's bespoke advice on fitness and nutrition made me stronger, feel positive, helped me sleep, and my back didn't hurt any more. And I never needed the hideous control underwear I'd bought to vacuum-pack my stomach in on my wedding day. Not then and not now, five years on.

"Now I have a daughter, Indy, who is two years old, and I want her to enjoy food without the hang-ups I had. *The Feelgood Plan* is something we embrace as a family. It isn't about restriction, or punishing "cleanses". *The Feelgood Plan* is about being healthy and happy, being in tune with your body, enjoying the foods you love and making time for the exercise and rest that makes you feel amazing. I believe *The Feelgood Plan* will make you happy to be you.'

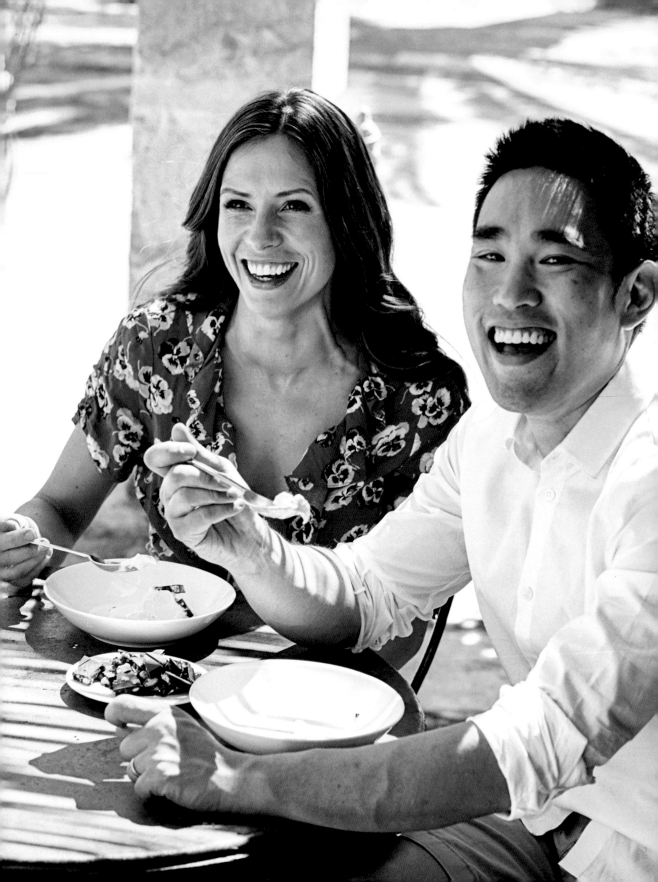

PART 1
START

1

Happy is just a few healthy steps away. You're going to start feeling better, right from this very moment. When you give your body what you need to feel your best, you'll want to do it all the time

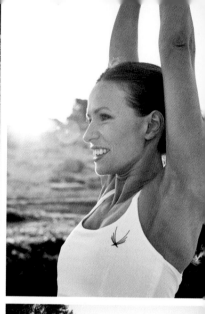

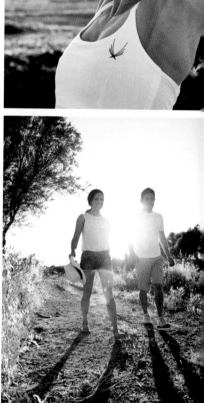

START FEELING GOOD 1

Healthy is happy. And the secret to feeling good is simple: tune into what your body needs

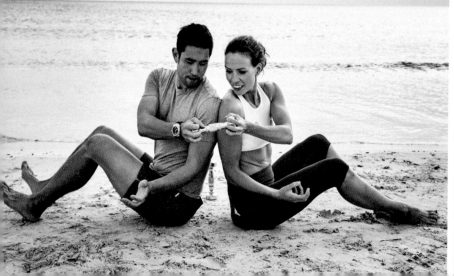

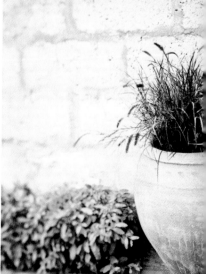

YOUR FIVE FEELGOOD GUIDELINES
This formula will help you understand what makes you feel good and will give you the power to make positive changes.

1 Take at least 15 minutes a day to put yourself first
Because looking after your body impacts everything. You're not just making healthy choices for your waistline, you're doing it because it means you have more energy for fun times, more patience with your loved ones and more brainpower at work. Making feelgood choices will improve your home life, work life and whole life.

2 Plan and eat proper, satisfying meals
Your key ingredients are protein, vegetables and complex carbs. Snacking is usually a gateway to overeating.

3 No foods are off-limits, but only eat when you're hungry
Stop when you're full. If you're not hungry, food isn't going to make you feel better.

4 You don't have to deprive yourself: there is always a feelgood option
It's totally possible to be healthy and have a life. So yes to burgers, chocolate and nights out.

5 When you're tired, you can get more energy from exercise or simply chiling out
Sugar isn't the solution.

Take at least 15 minutes a day for yourself. It's only 1% of your day: it's worth dedicating that time to look after number one

The Feelgood Plan is a happy, healthy way of life. It's a method for making everything you do a little bit easier, a fraction happier. It's how to shake off symptoms that grind us down, like fatigue, bloating, colds, weight gain and skin flare-ups. These are your body's cries for help. It's the physical drama-queen way of tossing its tiara across the room and shouting, "I need some support here! I have repairs to do! Can I please eat some vitamins at lunchtime? I need to stretch these stressed-out shoulders! And if I don't get decent sleep tonight, I will kick up seven shades of crazy!"

So when you give your body the foods, exercise and rest it needs, the complaints hush up, those unhappy symptoms vanish and you feel good. That's when you've got the energy to enjoy late nights, the metabolism to burn up pizza and chocolate and the strength to love challenging your body with exercise. When you're in the feelgood zone, you are your happiest, smartest, most easy-going version of yourself.

But if you ignore what your body's trying to tell you, that stressed, tired feeling simply won't shake. ODing on late nights, unhealthy foods and the sofa will eventually make you feel tired, bloated and run-down.

Why do your emotions matter?
Because they're what sabotage your intentions to exercise and eat well.

Here's where using the mood curve on the next page can help you get into the feelgood zone. This high-and-low flow may happen over a month, a week or even a day. For example, perhaps you had a big week and by Friday night you're exhausted. That's when you use your intuition (with a little help from this book) to choose the right foods, exercise and relaxation to lift yourself up to the feelgood zone for your week ahead. As you start to feel the benefits of eating and exercising intuitively, you'll instinctively make more healthy choices to stay at the top of the curve.

There's no desperate detox week or brutal bootcamp regime in this book—it's all about making small changes to get big results. Perhaps in the past you've tried to make drastic changes to your lifestyle and become overwhelmed and exhausted. But the scientifically proven way to achieve a big goal is to scale up to it gently [1]. Just 15 minutes to prepare a healthy meal, exercise or simply take time out makes a big difference. Remember, that's just 1% of your day. You see how small choices have a big impact on your body and when those choices are easy, or become ingrained habits, you have more willpower and you see more opportunities to feel even better.

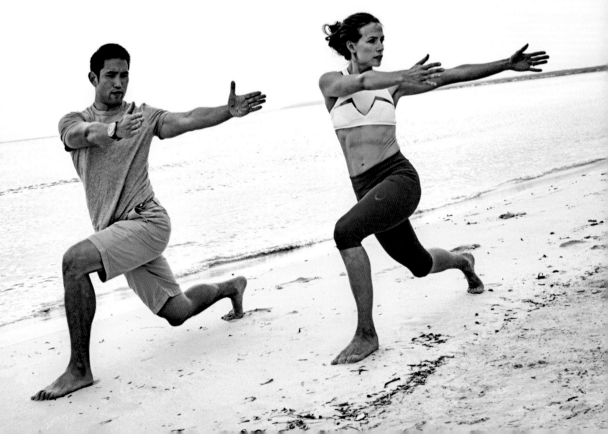

How do you feel today?
Answer the questions below to pinpoint
your position on the mood curve

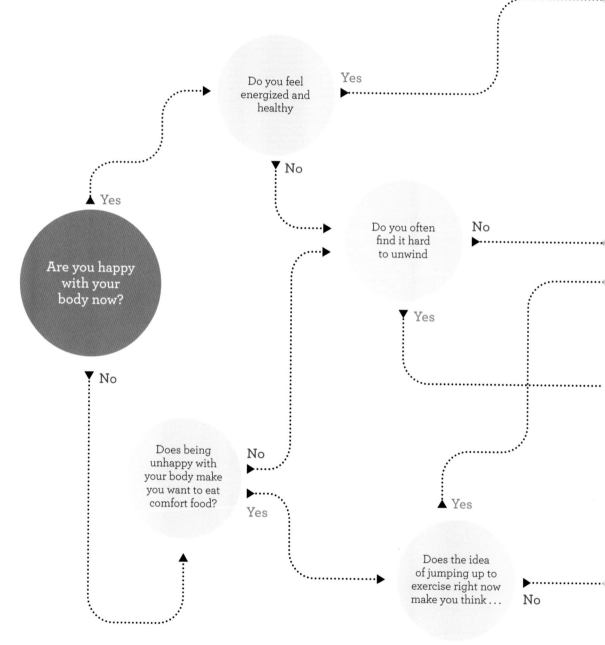

Are you happy
with your
body now?

▲ Yes

▼ No

Do you feel
energized and
healthy

Yes

▼ No

Do you often
find it hard
to unwind

No

▼ Yes

Does being
unhappy with
your body make
you want to eat
comfort food?

No

Yes

▲ Yes

Does the idea
of jumping up to
exercise right now
make you think . . .

▶ No

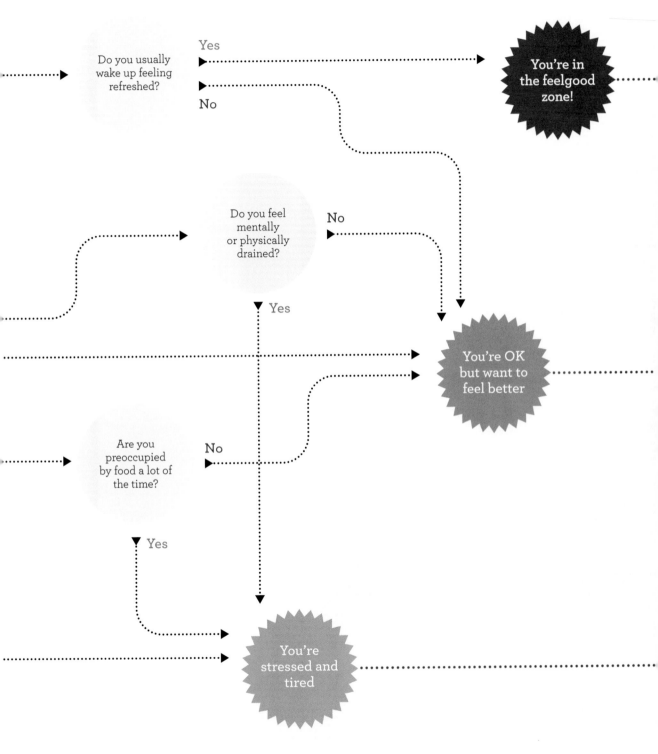

Do you usually wake up feeling refreshed?

Yes

No

You're in the feelgood zone!

Do you feel mentally or physically drained?

No

Yes

You're OK but want to feel better

Are you preoccupied by food a lot of the time?

No

Yes

You're stressed and tired

YOUR ROUTE TO THE FEELGOOD ZONE WHEN YOU'RE STRESSED AND TIRED

Take one small step

Why are you feeling low? Because you're not happy with the way things are. Why aren't you happy with the status quo? Because it doesn't make you feel good. Lows are your body's way of forcing you to make a positive change and regenerate. Making healthy choices is proven to make you feel emotionally stronger and happier [2]. Start with the very next thing you put in your mouth.

Nourish your body

When you try to fight the lows by eating junk food, you end up feeling worse. If you gorge on cake and other carb-laden treats when you feel bad, the insulin crash afterwards sinks your mood even lower. Eating the right vitamins, minerals, protein, fat and carbohydrates mean your body and brain can function at their very best.
In Eat, you'll find a nourishing menu of meals and snacks.

Zap fatigue with gentle exercise

It might seem contradictory to lace your trainers up when you want to lie on the sofa, but people who do 15 minutes of moderate exercise, like a brisk walk or cycle ride, feel a 65% boost in energy [3].
Reclaim your youthful bounce with the easy Anti-Ager workout (page 130).

Stretch away pain

Aching shoulders, backs, stomachs and, oh, *everything* are all part of feeling stressed. But low-intensity exercise triggers the release of pain-relieving endorphins and meditation can make colds history.
Try the headache-healing stretches (page 174) to start going up on the mood curve.

Get a good night's sleep

When you're feeling low, you need more sleep to regenerate your body.
If you don't sleep well, read the 3-minute sleep trick (page 182) that makes you wake refreshed.

WHEN YOU'RE IN THE FEELGOOD ZONE, YOU CAN...

Enjoy cake guilt-free

There's no, "Oooh, I shouldn't," about it: at the top of the curve, you've earned the right to enjoy every mouthful of cake because you've got the metabolism to burn it off. What's more, people who associate cake with guilt are more likely to gain weight than those who link it with a celebration [4]. So if you crave a slice, really enjoy it. The happier you are, and the fitter you are, the more treats you can have without feeling the strain on your waistband or the sluggishness in your step. Goodbye anxiety.

Swerve hangovers

Another bonus to feeling fit and happy: your hangovers will feel less hellish. How come? Because when your body is working at 100% capacity, your liver can process alcohol quicker.
Check out page 108 for the feelgood guide to drinking.

Leave the office on time

Feeling good makes you 12% more productive [5], and when you skip away from your desk with bags of energy for a good evening, you feel even better.

Set a new PB

When you're in a positive mental state, your body is more receptive to high-intensity exercise. Now is the time to challenge your body—you can push yourself without smashing through the pain barrier and getting injured.
Are you ready? Turn to the Power Circuits on page 150

Burn the candle at both ends

In the feelgood zone, you have boundless energy and your body needs less time to repair, so you can function with a little less sleep.
Uncover the secret life of your sleeping body on page 181.

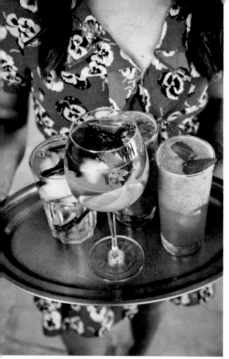
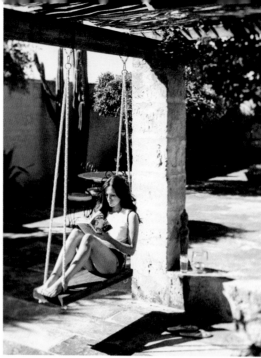
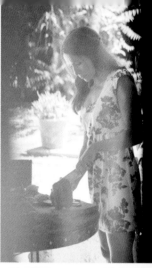
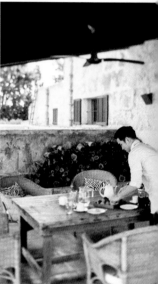

CHANGE YOUR BODY WITH YOUR MIND 2

Your approach to life *directly* affects how you look and feel. Here's how to set your mind to a happier, fitter you

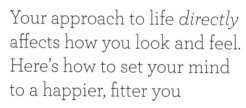
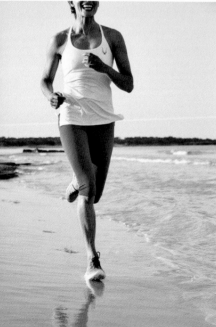
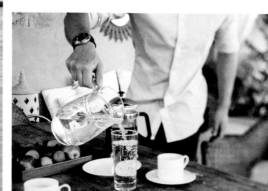
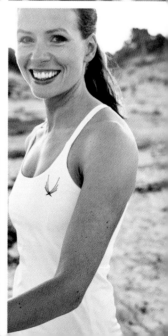

Doing the right thing for your body makes you feel good. But if it were that simple you would have done it already. No one purposely sets out to feel bloated, to get a headache or toss and turn all night.

Master the art of listening to your body and you'll put an end to creeping weight gain and other pesky issues before they escalate into something more serious. But when you're not so healthy, it's tricky to understand what your body is trying to tell you.

Our heads play host to a lot of conflicting chatter, which make us grab quick-fixes to make us feel better.

Ice cream will stop you feeling sad

You'll feel better if you have a cookie. Hey, finish the sleeve

Chips and wine, then you'll feel fine

Stressy morning? Have a croissant

And some of it can be pretty cruel…

Everyone thinks you eat cupcakes all day, so you may as well have a few

You may as well scoff down that bacon cheese-burger, you're fat anyway

You're too busy! Who do you think you are, taking time for yourself?

You're never going to look good in a bikini, what does it matter if you pig out?

Negative thoughts like these quickly generate an emotional response that you physically feel in your body:

Your shoulders creep up around your ears, dialling your stress up even more and you need to eat chocolate to soothe that tension

Your stomach knots and you reach for French fries to smother the discomfort

You almost hold your breath and want to distract yourself with something pleasant, like chips

You want to shut the stress down, so you instinctively reach for a massive glass of wine, like an emotional tranquillizer

In the moment, with all that going on in your body, you feel under pressure to grab a familiar treat, like sweets, chips or chocolate, hoping it will make you feel better. But the usual sugar-addled, highly processed foods we reach for ultimately make us feel worse. Studies show that in the present we're hyperaware of our feelings [1] but we struggle to do things in the now, like eat healthily, that benefit us in the future [2]. What's more, we often get hung up on trying to eat the right things and forget how to eat in a way that's right for us. We'll only feel better long-term when we tune in to what our bodies are really trying to tell us. That's when we do the right thing because we *want* to, not because we *have* to.

Wanting to look slimmer or to have clear skin aren't concerns that should be dismissed as a matter of vanity.
It doesn't make you shallow if you feel acne or weight gain chipping away at your confidence.

You deserve to feel good.
Be kind to yourself. Be kind
to your body. Look after it
and it will look after you.

If you're anything like 99.9% of people, you think of your future self as someone completely separate from the person sitting here, reading this book right now. Even though that future you is only weeks away. That person is someone you know pretty well already, but they're a happier, smarter version of you. They're more chilled out, yet more successful, too.

Your feelgood voice will help you connect to that future you right now. Take a step back, if only for a minute. Let everything else going on slide into silence. Listen: how do you want to feel?

How do you know that what you're listening to is your feelgood voice? Because it comes from your gut—you don't just hear it, you feel it resonate. The feelgood voice connects your body and mind. It makes sense. It wants the best for you.

Here's the clincher...

You have to want to feel good for yourself, or it won't resonate deep enough to motivate you over any bumps along the way. Your reason could be aesthetic ("I want to look good naked"), fundamental ("I want to have more energy with my kids"), emotional ("I want to stop feeling so stressed") or maybe it's a medical issue ("I want to stay healthy and not get sick like my dad"). At the moments when you falter, that is the anchor that will keep you steady. Write your reason here:

I want

and I *know* it will make me feel good

When you hear your negative voice creeping in, demanding not just one doughnut but a whole tray, go back to this anchor and find strength of mind. This practice will help you stop overeating and make healthier choices.

 Take 15 minutes to decide your reason and write it in the box above. Give it careful thought— when your resolve falters, you'll stay firm

THREE HABITS THAT HELP YOU BECOME EFFORTLESSLY HEALTHY AND HAPPY
No matter what hurdles you're up against, trust this trio to help you hop over them

It's taken over 40 years for geneticists to work out the key traits that determine how often you exercise, how well you eat and how much you look after yourself, and the results are gold [8]. The truth is that your attitude trumps genes: personality is intrinsically linked to being overweight, having high cholesterol and abnormally high blood pressure. So how can you be one of those slim, sorted people?

1 You plan
When you say you're going to exercise, you actually do. In fact, you book workouts into your diary as you would a board meeting, and treat them with the same respect. Your life is structured so eating healthily is easy— groceries are delivered regularly so your fridge is always stocked with fresh vegetables, you schedule time to cook nourishing meals, you plan what you're going to have for lunch tomorrow and your gym kit is packed, ready to go.

3 You're kind to yourself
If you eat well 80% of the time, then you deserve to use that 20% to enjoy pizza or a glass of wine without beating yourself up. There's no need to be super-strict. Focusing on your positives makes you kinder to yourself. You deserve to be looked after, to wake up feeling refreshed and to enjoy dessert without counting calories.

2 You pay attention
Guess what? When you're in tune with your body, you get a good idea of what you need to feed it so it functions at its best. Listening to your feelgood voice makes you naturally self-disciplined in an easy-going, non-obsessive way.

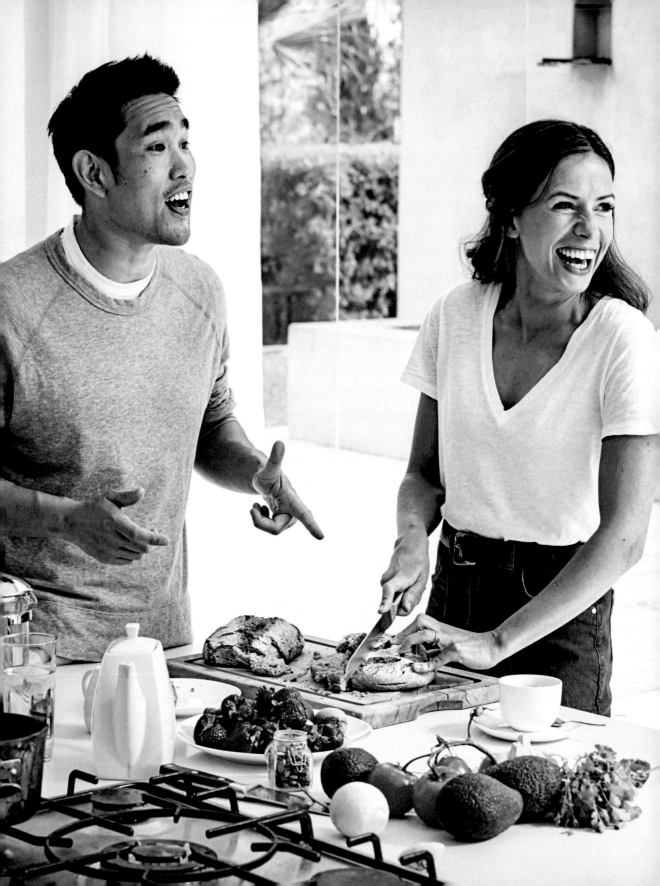

PART
EAT

2

Here's your go-to guide for exactly what to eat to satisfy your head, heart and hotpants. If you've ever worried about your weight before, you'll be relieved to know you can be a happy, healthy size without giving up all the fun stuff. It takes very little effort to look and feel amazing

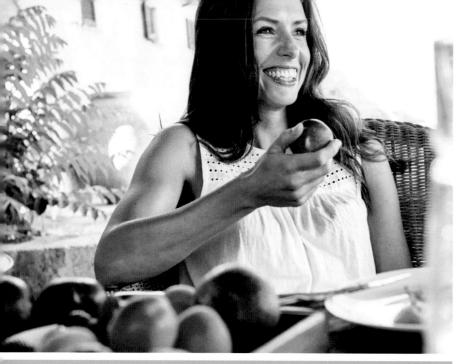

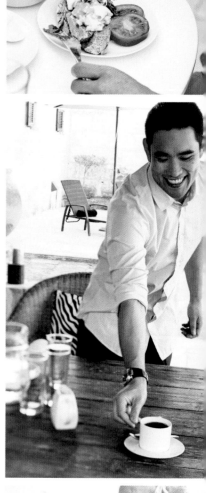

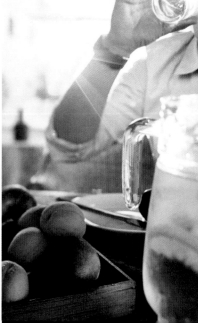

HOW HUNGRY ARE YOU REALLY? 3

Read your internal body language and discover when to eat, what to do when you've overdone it, and how to build a healthy relationship with food

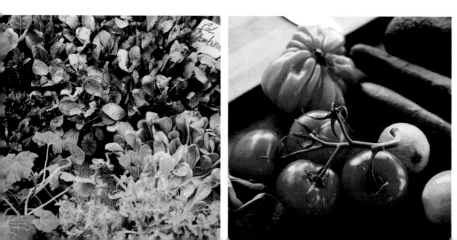

To understand hunger, it is essential to separate your need for nutrients from the desire to eat

In fact, how much you eat has little to do with how hungry you really are. How many times have you felt literally sick to the stomach by how much you've consumed? How often have you looked at an exquisite cupcake or a plate of fries and thought, "I don't need that, but I'm going to eat it anyway'? How frequently do you snack out of habit, and not because you have a real physical need for food?

Tuning into your hunger has huge benefits for your body. Obviously, when you only eat the food your body needs, you'll get the right nutrients and won't store excess fat or be overweight. Not only will understanding your hunger help you drop a size or two, but you could:

Skyarugula your sex drive: Trimming 10% off your body weight boosts satisfaction between the sheets [1].

Look younger: Losing weight has the effect of widening your eyes, sharpening your profile and making your skin glow—three key characteristics of youth.

Actually be younger: Dropping even a few pounds can lower your blood pressure and reduce the risk of serious problems like heart disease, diabetes and cancer, which all increase with age [2].

Get a promotion: If you are also a woman, that is. Slim women typically earn more than their overweight sisters (annoyingly, men aren't subject to the same discrimination) [3].

Crucially, getting a handle on hunger takes the stress out of food. Since eating is something we need to do several times a day, that cuts a huge amount of stress out of your life.

Your mood has a clear correlation with your ability to understand your true hunger signals. This chapter will help you ID hunger for exactly what it is: a physical need to nourish your body. Take a look at the mood curve overleaf to see how your mood messes with your hunger.

How does your attitude to food affect your mood?

Aha, so *that's* what's going on …

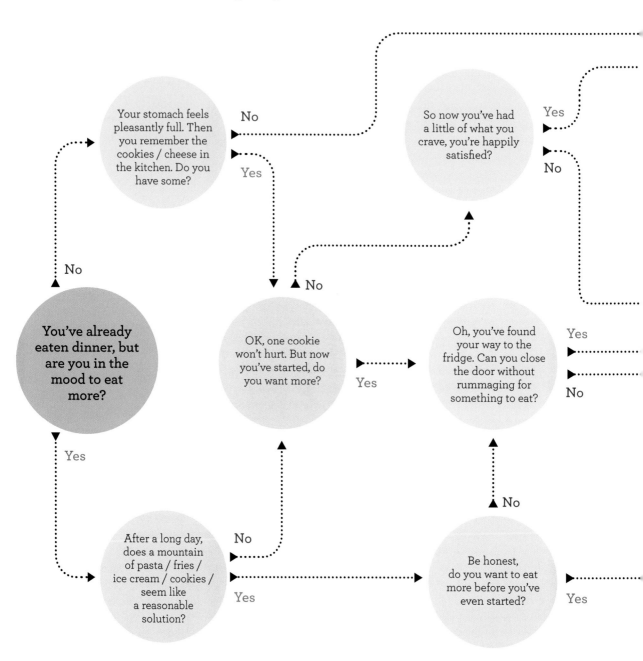

Your stomach feels pleasantly full. Then you remember the cookies / cheese in the kitchen. Do you have some?

No

Yes

So now you've had a little of what you crave, you're happily satisfied?

Yes

No

You've already eaten dinner, but are you in the mood to eat more?

No

Yes

OK, one cookie won't hurt. But now you've started, do you want more?

Yes

No

Oh, you've found your way to the fridge. Can you close the door without rummaging for something to eat?

Yes

No

No

After a long day, does a mountain of pasta / fries / ice cream / cookies / seem like a reasonable solution?

No

Yes

Be honest, do you want to eat more before you've even started?

Yes

No

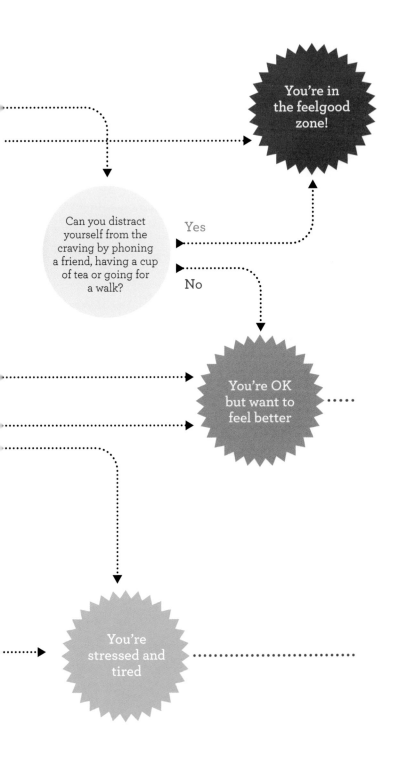

Can you distract yourself from the craving by phoning a friend, having a cup of tea or going for a walk?

Yes

No

You're in the feelgood zone!

You're OK but want to feel better

You're stressed and tired

Eat your way up the mood curve

We want to feel good. We don't want to feel tired, weighed down or uncomfortable after eating. But even though we know the foods that promise an immediate high also come with a kick-in-the-guts low, we still crave them. And by eating a mountainous muffin or a bucket of greasy chicken, we get further away from feeling good.

Self-sabotage happens because we fear change. When we're afraid, we convince ourselves we're going to slip up anyway, so why not bury your face in that cream cheese icing? That's the negative voice talking, not your truth-telling feelgood voice. It's time to get on your own team.

It may be a big change for you to eat healthily. It takes commitment. It's not as simple as waving a magic wand over your plate. To change your body, you have to change a few patterns.

At some level, you may realize your habits make you feel bad, but you're resistant to change because you don't know what else to do. The pain is familiar and a recognisable ache is easier to deal with than the unknown. But to stop stress-eating doesn't mean you'll stop coping with stress. So try other stress-reducing strategies, ones that won't undermine your ability to feel good and be the person you want to be. See the nutrition tips in this section and discover how exercise can be relaxing (page 138) and try wiggling away stress with a tennis ball (yes, you read that right) on page 170.

SEVEN WAYS TO SATISFY YOUR HUNGER
Your body is ready. Let's get cracking

1 Eat when you're calm
Eating while stressed can make it more difficult for your body to absorb vitamins and minerals, which means you're not getting goodness from your food. Rapid, stressed-out eating leads to bloating, gas, stomach cramps and diarrhea. Nice! It can also make you overeat, as you push food into your mouth so fast that you don't realize you're full before your waistband cuts painfully into your stomach. When you know you're feeling hangry (that's so hungry, you're angry), calm down before you eat by kneading the fleshy part between your thumb and forefinger for 30 seconds. Even a short hand massage lowers your heart rate and lessens anxiety [4].

2 Align your eyes with your stomach
We tend to serve portions according to how big our plates are, not how hungry we are. Break this habit by serving yourself two-thirds of your normal portion—you can always have the rest if you need more, but chances are this will be enough to satisfy your hunger.

3 Express gratitude for your food
Give thanks for what you are about to devour and your meal will taste better and feel more satisfying in every way. Out loud, observe the colors and delicious textures of your food, and thank the cook (especially if it's you). Internally, pay attention to the ways your meal will nourish your body: think about how that roast beef will give you iron strength, or how the vitamin C in your blueberries will help you feel calmer.

4 Chew, chew, chew
Chewing releases more nutrients from food. Start munching at least ten times before you swallow and work up to doubling that number. Slim people chew each mouthful an average of twenty-one times [5]. Breaking down food in your mouth like this helps your stomach signal fullness to your brain more quickly.

5 Eat in slo-mo
Place your knife and fork down between mouthfuls to break the hand-to-mouth flow when you eat. If you're right-handed, try eating with your left, and vice versa, to help slow your pace.

6 Eat with all of your senses

This trick stops you filling up on so-so food that gives you little physical or emotional satisfaction. How does your food look? How does it smell? Note its texture and the sound it makes as you chew. Appreciating your food means you get more enjoyment from eating, and it slows your mealtime down so your body has time to recognize when you are full.

7 Prioritize your plate

Your mom's not watching, and there's no law that says you have to finish everything on your plate. You can only comfortably fit so much in your stomach, so fill it up with healthy foods like vegetables and lean protein, and leave the extras that might make you feel painfully overfull.

Why you may need to eat MORE to LOSE weight
Yes, you read that correctly

If you're trying to lose weight, don't be tempted to starve yourself. When you don't give your body enough nutrients and energy to function, the first place your body goes to steal those nutrients from is your muscles. And when you don't have enough lean muscle, your body burns less fat. The fat stored around your hips, thighs, belly and upper arms is always the last place your body looks for nutrients, because fat is where toxins are stored. Want more proof? Low calorie consumption is proven to slow metabolism [6].

To shed fat, pile your plate with the three powerhouses. First, vegetables. These are crucial because they are packed with nutrients, low in calories, a good source of healthy complex carbohydrates and they use a lot of energy just to digest. Second, quality protein is essential because it helps repair your muscles and gives you clean energy. Thirdly, adding a little healthy fat to every meal helps you feel full for longer. With these nutritious foods on your menu, you can enjoy eating without taking on excess calories.

HOW OFTEN SHOULD YOU EAT?
Ask the right questions to find the right answer for you

Eating at regular intervals helps you maintain a healthy weight [7]. It doesn't matter whether you eat every three hours or stick to three meals a day as long as you have a regular pattern and are aware of how much you're consuming each time you eat.

To find the pattern that works for you, experiment with having somewhere between three and six meals a day. Then ask yourself:

Q: Can you make time to stop what you're doing and eat?
If not, then eat less often, but eat bigger meals. Give your food 100% attention and it will satisfy you more.

Q. Does eating every few hours feel like you're eating pretty much constantly?
If you're grazing all day, space your meals out and make each one more substantial, otherwise you'll give your body far more food than it needs.

Q: Are you hungry enough between meals that you feel ready to eat?
If not, then spread your meals out further.

Q. Do you get so hungry before a meal that you just want to grab something convenient that gives you instant energy?
If so, eat more often as this will help you make smart food choices.

Q. Do you feel satisfied after your meal?
If not, you're spreading your calories too thin. Try eating bigger meals less often.

Q. Are you giving your body steady energy throughout the day?
You're doing just right.

TIP If you increase meal frequency, decrease meal size, so whether you eat three, four, five or six times a day, the total amount is the same.

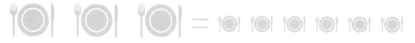

Maintaining a healthy weight ultimately comes down to how much you consume over the course of the day [8].

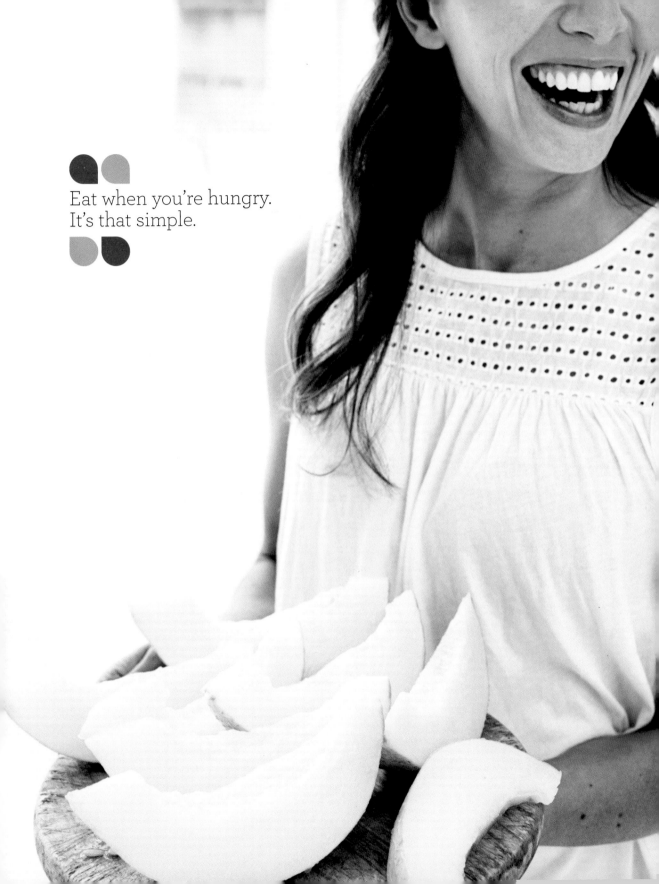

Eat when you're hungry.
It's that simple.

HOW TO STOP OVEREATING

Fifteen minutes. That's how long it takes for your stomach to let your brain know that it is stuffed. But you can throw a lot of food down the hatch in 15 minutes. Avoid that uncomfortably-full feeling by asking yourself these three questions:

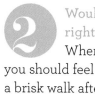 **If you stop now, would you be satisfied?**
When you've eaten half the food on your plate, lay your cutlery down and pause for 10 seconds. Would another bite be satisfying or uncomfortable? Looking out for your "Aha!" moment makes you more mindful of how your stomach feels.

Is it December 25th today? Thanksgiving? Hanukkah? The end of Ramadan?
Consider the difference between feeling pleasantly full and once-a-year-stuffed. If your stomach is pushing towards turkey-and-stuffing territory, you're done. It's time to lay down your fork and get up from the table.

 Would a walk in the park right now be nice?
When you're pleasantly full, you should feel able to get up and go for a brisk walk after your meal and not feel weighed down. You should have more energy after eating, not so little you need to lie down.

Hunger [huhng-ger]
noun: a compelling need for food
verb: to have a strong desire

> **Allow 15 minutes for your belly to let your brain know whether you're genuinely hungry—you may discover you're actually full**

OUCH! WHAT TO DO WHEN YOU'VE EATEN TOO MUCH
Take this quick quiz to reveal your recovery remedy

How does your stomach feel?

A You've got a sudden blow-out bloat
B Something is sitting heavily in your gut

You're craving something. What is it?

A Cheese
B Sugar

What's going on in your head?

A You feel jittery and a headache is brewing
B You feel sleepy and slow

If you answered mostly As:
you ate too many sugary carbohydrates

YOUR CARB OVERDOSE RECOVERY PLAN:

Bring your insulin down by eating a little healthy fat and protein. Try a slice of hand-carved turkey with some avocado on top.

Fennel is excellent for evening out blood sugar. It takes just 10 minutes for the fiber in these green bulbs to boost energy and slow glucose production in your liver [9].

Sip extra water, as carbohydrates absorb H20 in your stomach, so you need extra fluids to move it through your gut and avoid constipation.

Light exercise, like a gentle stroll or some slow yoga, will help contract your digestive muscles and break down the excess of carbs. Tomorrow, your muscles will be full of glycogen, so you can bust through a high-intensity workout—may as well put those carbs to good use.

If you answered mostly Bs:
you overate fats and protein

YOUR PROTEIN AND FAT OVERDOSE RECOVERY PLAN:

Eat pineapple, which is high in an enzyme called bromelain that can help your body break down protein.

Drink tea or coffee, as the caffeine will give you a kick of energy. It stimulates your adrenal glands to help you process the protein.

Eat a handful of raw nuts and seeds, as these are high in lipase, the enzyme that breaks down fats.

Take a digestive enzyme supplement to break down the protein so it won't sit heavily in your gut for long.

THE HEALTHY, HAPPY WAY
TO GUARANTEE WEIGHT LOSS
It's right here in front of you

You don't need a rigid, aggressive diet to lose weight. By following the 12-week feelgood plan on pages 186–213, you'll fine-tune your body and get results that last forever. What's more, you'll feel happy and energized as you do it. To help you feel tuned in to your body, start by keeping a food diary. It's scientifically proven that a food diary is the best way to monitor your eating habits without becoming obsessive [10]. Keep it quick and easy—try something like this:

When did you eat?

What did you eat?

Did you enjoy your food?

How did you feel at the time?

How did you feel afterwards?

As you fill out your diary, you may find yourself making better choices. Great! But it's just as important to acknowledge your mistakes, because being honest will help you be in tune with body. You will take missteps: you're human. The more aware you are of how your eating habits make you feel, the better you'll treat your body. After a few days, you'll see a pattern emerging. Once you know what the problem is, you can refer to the relevant pages in this book to work out a solution.

Looks too much like effort? Keep a photographic food diary instead. Use your smartphone to snap everything you eat before it goes into your mouth—yup, even the swig of orange juice you sneak as you open the fridge door. Picture diaries can be even more effective than written ones because "they serve as intervention at the point when decisions regarding what to eat are being made" [11]. In English? The act of photographing your food can stop you mindlessly consuming more than you need. Do whatever works for you.

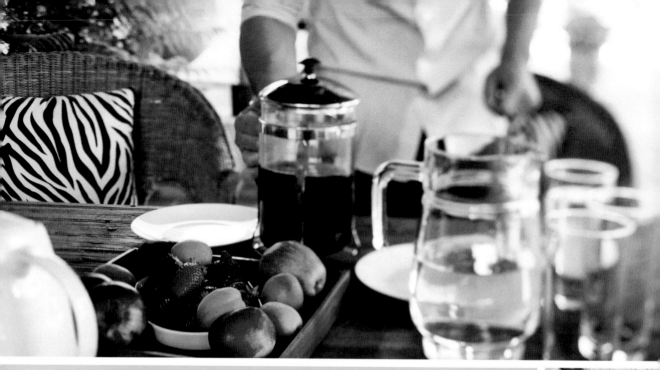

THE FEELGOOD GUIDE TO BREAKFAST 4

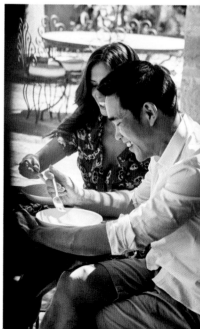

Having a superpowered start is the foundation for feeling good all day long

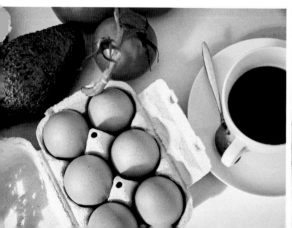

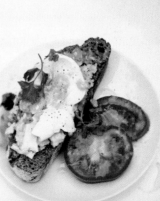

So simple when you think about it: when breakfast makes you feel good, you have the energy to enjoy everything life throws at you today. What's more, you eat better for the next 24 hours and discover superhuman snack-sidestepping willpower

Take advantage of the fact that your metabolism is most efficient in the morning. People who eat a large breakfast and a light dinner typically lose two-and-a-half times more weight than those who eat a small breakfast and a big dinner [1].

Variety is the key to getting all the nutrients you need. Experiment with the feelgood grid on the next page and mix up your menu. Pancakes, smoked salmon, blueberries with creamy Greek yogurt—they're all good.

Eggs are the most filling breakfast [2]. They only take 3 minutes to cook—or even faster if you keep a bowl of beaten eggs in the fridge, ready to go.

Sneak greens into your breakfast by adding asparagus to poached eggs or throwing last night's sautéed veggies into an omelette. If you don't likeeating vegetables in the morning, blend a green juice and drink them instead.

If breakfast isn't breakfast for you unless it involves toast and cereal, choose the feelgood options and add protein. Try scrambled eggs on rye or oatmeal with a scoop of protein powder.

Watch out for hidden sugar, as it sets you up for a mid-morning slump. Muffins and pastries are obvious no-nos, but sugar also lurks in 90% of processed foods, including ketchup, granola, flavored yogurt and orange juice.

Want a healthy sweet fix? Chop strawberries into cereal or grate apple into your granola. Fresh fruit beats juice or dried fruit every time as you get more flavor, more fiber and less sugar.

We're all dehydrated in the morning; 8 hours without fluids makes us sluggish. Have a big glass of water by your bed for when you wake up and another with your breakfast. Within 10 minutes of rehydrating, your metabolic rate rises 30%.

Allow 1% of your day to prepare a healthy breakfast, then sit down and eat it

START YOUR DAY THE FEELGOOD WAY

FEELS BAD	FEELS OK	FEELS GOOD

On the go

Breakfast bar—what is this bar stuck together with? The answer is sugar. That's why it sates your hunger for a mere 10 minutes. Bars for breakfast won't make you feel good for long

Protein shake—nourishes your body, especially if you buy protein powder made from organic whey, as it won't contain pesticides or chemicals. Unflavored powders have less sugar—add a healthy burst of sweetness by blending your shake with a handful of frozen berries and some almond milk

Green juice—try our feelgood go-to: ginger, lemon, cucumber, spinach, celery and a dollop of nut butter. Add an apple, berries or half a banana if you like yours sweeter, plus a scoop of protein powder to make it feel like more of a meal. Have the ingredients ready in the blender so all you do in the morning is push a button

Breakfast bowls

Granola, yogurt and compote—a staple of coffee shops, this is a bowl of sugar masquerading as a healthy breakfast. Granola is muesli covered in sugar, while "compote" is a posh name for "jam"

Classic granola muesli—this summery version of oatmeal doesn't quite live up to its healthy intentions, thanks to the fact it's made by soaking oats in sugar-laced apple juice and served with huge handfuls of dried fruit, which contain concentrated sugar

Berry smoothie bowl—blend a few handfuls of fresh or frozen raspberries and blueberries with half a banana, half an avocado, a big teaspoon of coconut oil and a scoop of protein powder. Top with nuts and more berries

Bread

White bread—eating a mere 120g of white bread a day can cause obesity [3]. Why? It's processed sugar. If you have to eat white bread, buy the freshly baked variety, slice it at home and freeze. It toasts fine from frozen and doesn't have the toxic preservatives of processed white bread

Wholegrain bread with seeds—complex carbs slowly release energy thanks to their natural fiber, so you stay full for longer

Dark, heavy breads like rye and spelt—in addition to the wholegrain benefits, nutty-tasting dark breads are rich in magnesium, which can reduce your risk of type 2 diabetes

FEELS BAD	FEELS OK	FEELS GOOD

Spreads

Margarine—synthetic gunk loaded with additives. Without colorings, margarine is actually grey

Butter—it's high in vitamin A, which is vital for a healthy immune system, cell growth and good vision. The link between butter's natural saturated fat and heart disease is pure fiction [4]—the urban myth was spread by manipulative margarine manufacturers

Organic butter—all the vitamins and minerals of butter, without any traces of chemicals and pesticides

Toast toppings

Jam or marmalade—they're just sugar. If you can't imagine life without jam, have a home-made one instead as it will only contain natural preservatives

Natural peanut butter—eating PB in the morning is proven to raise your levels of peptide YY, the "thank you, I'm full" hormone. Peanut butter also helps control cravings for up to 12 hours afterwards [5]. But a word of caution: non-organic PB is high in pesticides and fungus and contains aflatoxin, a potential carcinogen. Put your peanut butter in the fridge to slow down its growth

Organic nut butters—one of the most important products to buy organic, because fat easily absorbs and retains pesticides, and nuts are fat. Eating a variety of nut butters means you get a range of vitamins and minerals: heart-healthy oleic acid from cashews; vitamin E from almonds; calcium and iron from peanuts; and walnut butter is one of the best vegetarian sources of omega-3 fatty acids

Cereal

Sugary cereals—not just frosted flakes, we're talking granola, cornflakes covered in honey and even muesli packed with dried fruit. If you must, choose a brand with large flakes—it means you'll consume fewer calories without noticing the difference [6]

Bran-based cereals and nutty muesli—less sugary than those on the left, but the third ingredient of bran flakes is still sugar. Measure a half-cup portion so you don't accidentally overeat and give yourself a groaning stomach

Bespoke-blend granola—grate half an apple into a bowl and mix in 2 tbsp of oats, 1 tsp chia seeds, plus a handful each of blueberries and almonds. Cover with whole milk and leave overnight; in the morning you have a sweet and satisfying brekkie

FEELS BAD	FEELS OK	FEELS GOOD

Oatmeal

Instant oatmeal—salt and sugar are often added by the manufacturer, while the whole grain is taken out so you won't stay full for long

Home-made oatmeal—high in fiber, which reduces bad cholesterol and helps you stay full for longer. Add a pinch of cinnamon or nutmeg on top for a sweeter, spicier taste

Home-made oatmeal with organic steel-cut oats—also known as "Irish oats', this variety is lower on the glycaemic index than rolled oats, so it helps to stabilize your blood sugar. Soak your oats in milk overnight so they cook in just one minute in the morning

Milk

Skim or 1% cows' milk—vitamin A, essential for good vision and a robust immune system, occurs naturally in milk, but it requires fat to be used by the body. So skimming off the fat isn't the healthy option

Whole cows' milk—whole milk typically contains 50% more omega-3 fatty acids than 1% and 66% more than skim milk

Organic whole cows' milk, oat milk, rice milk, coconut milk or almond milk—organic milk is free from the pesticides and chemicals in commercial farming. Organic cows' milk delivers 62% more healthy omega-3 fats [7]: good news for your heart. Try making your oatmeal with rice, almond or coconut milk to get a variety of nutrients

Fruit

Pre-packed tropical fruit salad—pre-cut fruit often contains a fraction of the vitamin C it would have had when fresh [8]. Packaged fruit is often cut up abroad for cost reasons, so it has to be chemically treated to maintain the appearance of freshness. If you love tropical fruit, chop it yourself to preserve the nutrients. Eat it with a handful of raw nuts to slow down the sugar kick

Small fruit salad—though this looks healthy, it is unlikely to fill you up so you'll probably want a snack before lunch. Make yours properly satisfying by adding Greek yogurt, nuts and seeds to a variety of fruit. We like pear, apple and berries, which have plenty of color and stomach-soothing fiber, too

Big bowl of blueberries, strawberries, raspberries and blackberries—berries are packed with flavorsome antioxidants and immune-boosting phytonutrients. These fruits are relatively low in sugar and their intense colors prove they are bursting with nutrients. A handful of berries is fine if you're having protein pancakes or Greek yogurt too, but if not then be generous because a small bowl of berries probably won't power you through to lunch. Eat your fruit with a sprinkle of almonds and pumpkin seeds, too

FEELS BAD	FEELS OK	FEELS GOOD

Yogurt

Fruit on the bottom yogurt—sugar with a side of sugar. That explains why you could eat three in one morning

Low-fat yogurt and flavored yogurt—when manufacturers remove the fat, they replace it with sugar. And fruity flavorings offer negligible nutritional benefits, they're just sugar. That extra sugar triggers cravings so over the day you're likely to eat more

Whole-fat Greek yogurt—regularly eating full-fat yogurt can reduce the risk of obesity by 12% [9]. How so? It's thought the higher fat content stops you overeating. If dairy makes you bloated, try yummy coconut yogurt instead

Eggs

Fried eggs or eggs covered in hollandaise sauce—the unhealthiest way to eat eggs

Omelette or scrambled eggs—use fresh herbs like coriander or dill on top of your eggs to add flavor

Poached or boiled eggs—eggs are healthiest when untampered. A complete egg delivers the perfect balance of protein and healthy fat, and the yolk contains the most nutrients

Meat

Sausages or bacon—salt, nitrates and other chemicals added during processing are difficult to detox, so we store them in our fat cells, which means more cellulite. Eating processed red meat every day has also been linked to an increased risk of cancer

Organic sausages or bacon—though you're spared the worst of the processing horrors, pork eaten this way is still overly full of salt and fat. Cook just two sausages or strips of bacon so you're not tempted to snack on them later

Organic hand-carved ham – it's unprocessed, pesticide-free and as close to nature as possible, so it's a smart protein choice for breakfast. Ham tastes great with soft-boiled eggs and watercress—give it a go

Fish

Fish stick sandwich—white bread is high GI and fish sticks are often pre-fried before being frozen. Adding brown sauce or ketchup? More sugar

Home-made fish sticks on an open sandwich—brush a beaten egg over your fish fillets, roll them in breadcrumbs and you've got a more satisfying breakfast

Smoked salmon, kippers or mackerel—they're all good sources of omega-3 fatty acids, though smoked fish is high in salt so treat yourself just a few mornings a week

FEELS BAD	FEELS OK	FEELS GOOD

Pancakes

Instant pancake mix with squirty cream, maple syrup and icing sugar—fried sugar, synthetic creamy sugar, sticky sugar and dusty sugar

Home-made pancakes made with non-organic ingredients—it's OK, but you can go one better

Home-made, organic protein pancakes—blend 1 cup cottage cheese, 1 cup oats or rye flakes, four eggs and a generous shake of cinnamon. The mixture will last for up to three days in the fridge and the pancakes take two minutes each side in a medium hot pan

Fruit drinks

Orange juice—without the fruit's natural fiber, you're drinking a glass of sugar that gives you an insulin spike...and then a crash, even if it is freshly squeezed. If mornings without OJ aren't worth waking up for, smooth the spike by eating a high-fiber breakfast. Chia seeds have twice the fiber of bran flakes—try yours with yogurt

Fruit smoothie—blend yours with fresh or frozen fruits, a handful of ice and a spoonful of yogurt. The yogurt adds protein and the crushed ice gives the smoothie a satiating texture

Fresh lemon with water—though lemons are acidic, when you digest them you get an alkaline effect. Why does that matter? Because balancing the acidity of your blood can improve heart health, boost brain function, reduce back pain and lower your risk of obesity and colon cancer

Coffee

Instant coffee—the processed variety is high in acrylamide, a chemical compound that has been shown to cause cancer and nerve damage in animals. Acrylamide wasn't found in food until 2002, so scientists don't know the full risks yet

Ground coffee—the kind you buy from coffee shops or make using your at-home coffee machine gives you a caffeine buzz without the chemical headache

Organic ground coffee—an even better brew, as it doesn't contain any traces of pesticides or fungicides. It's literally ground coffee beans and hot water. Doctors recommend drinking no more than three cups a day, so why not drink the best quality?

Tea

English breakfast tea with sugar—getting stuck into the sweet stuff this early sets you on a rollercoaster insulin ride where your cravings are hard to control

Herbal tea—ginger tea curbs nausea, peppermint soothes stomach cramps, while milk thistle and dandelion are gentle liver cleansers. English breakfast tea is OK, too, as long as you stick to a splash of milk, no sugar

Green tea—this natural fat-burning drink is loaded with antioxidants that help protect your cells from damage and disease. It not only gives you a caffeine buzz, but also it contains the amino acid L-theanine, which improves brain function

Make your coffee count by drinking a cup when cortisol naturally dips in the day, so you feel more alert in an energy slump. Caffeine increases the production of cortisol, the stress hormone, so try waiting until after breakfast to have your first cup [10]. Around 10am is the perfect time.

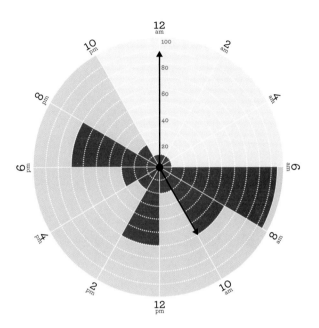

If the thought of breakfast makes you nauseous, your body is trying to tell you something.

Listen. If you don't feel hungry, it's crazy to force yourself to eat. It takes 4 days for your body to go into starvation mode and suppress metabolism, so a missed or mid-morning breakfast won't mess you up [11]. In fact, it will gently burn the fat stored on your hips, thighs and around your middle. Enjoy an extra 15 minutes in bed in the morning or get up and do some stretches, then eat when you're ready.

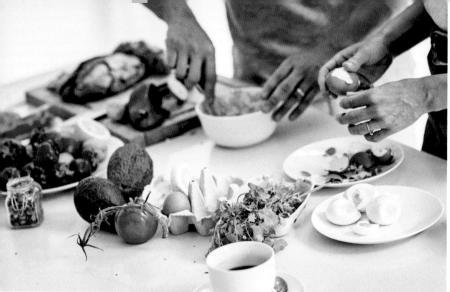

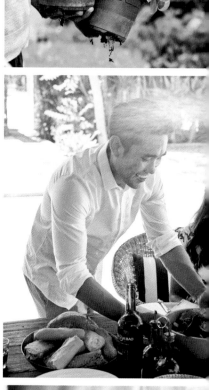

THE FEELGOOD GUIDE TO LUNCH 5

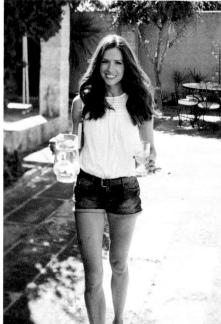

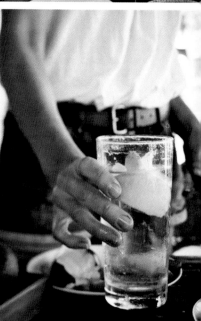

We make scores of important decisions every day, yet when it comes to choosing what to eat for lunch, we flounder—which inevitably leads to snacking in the afternoon. Here's your get-it-sorted guide

What makes the ultimate power lunch? It's your favorite go-to, with a few healthy tweaks to give you feelgood energy all afternoon

For zero lunch hour indecision tomorrow, save a portion of tonight's healthy dinner. A colorful heap of stir-fried vegetables and turkey holds well in your lunchbox, as does chili and moussaka. Box up with crunchy veggies like peppers, cucumber and sugar snap peas as these stay crisp. Homemade soups travel neatly, too. As well as saving money, packing a lunchbox is a good way to control portion size.

One simple trick for fuelling a busy afternoon without ransacking the cookie tin: eat a palm-sized portion of protein.

If you want to be slimmer, load a quarter of your plate with vegetables. They're so nourishing you end up consuming 350 fewer calories in the day.

Get outside to combat carb cravings— you know the white potato urge you get when you're tired? That. Walking also increases energising blood flow and stimulates digestion so your lunch won't sit heavily.

Lunch doesn't feel right without a sandwich? Then chew mindfully and you'll be so satisfied you won't need chips too. If you struggle to pace yourself, cut your sandwich into small pieces. Eating small bites can mean you eat less later on in the day without even thinking about it [1].

Cut out hidden sugar in energy drinks and fruit juice, and you can embrace a little out-and-out sugar without much impact on your waistline. People who exercise but enjoy a small sweet treat every day typically have a lower BMI than those who abstain [2]. So if you have a sweet tooth, finish your lunch with a few squares of dark chocolate.

If you know dinner isn't until 8pm, grab a healthy snack for the afternoon while you're getting lunch. Planning what to eat means you're more likely to choose a healthy option, like cashew butter and crackers, instead of whatever random cookies are lurking in the office.

Save 15 minutes of your lunch break to get outside. Fresh air and movement are far more energising than staying at your desk

LUNCHES FOR LASTING ENERGY

FEELS BAD	FEELS OK	FEELS GOOD

Salad

Pasta salad with mayo and croutons—too much unhealthy fat, way too much sodium and far too few nutrients. Say "no thanks" to potato salad and coleslaw for the same reasons. A mono-colored meal is a miserable one

Supermarket salad box with chicken, cous cous and a few vegetables—add some extra protein (a chicken breast, prawns or egg) and just use half the dressing to make this salad more satisfying

Home-made salad—with grilled chicken breast, avocado, egg, loads of colorful vegetables and different textures from pumpkin seeds, walnuts and sprouting shoots. Tasty, filling and packed with vitamins and minerals to power your day

Sandwich

White bread sandwich with bacon and mayo—you'll crash and want more within the hour

Open-facing sandwich on whole wheat bread—choose simple ingredients like ham, cheese or (mayo-free) tuna. The fewer, the better

No-bread sandwich—which is basically triple the protein and vegetable fillings, minus the high-GI bread

Soup

Creamy tinned soups—especially potato-based ones as they're simultaneously high in sodium, unhealthy fats and refined sugar. A nutrient-free bowl

Fresh carton of soup—opt for a vegetable blend because most meaty flavors aren't organic. If you like bread, dunk a hunk of dark rye

Home-made chicken broth or vegetable soup—a bowl can mean you eat 20% less for lunch [3]

Chicken

Fried chicken—in theory, chicken is a good meat to eat at lunch because it's easy to digest, but not when it's poor-quality chicken fried to hell and back. It has minimal nutritional content

Rotisserie chicken—an OK choice for lunch because you're getting plenty of protein, and you'll have plenty to eat later in the week. Skip the skin and eat your chicken with fresh spinach, radishes for crunch and peppers for texture and colorful sweetness

Organic roast chicken—prime, nourishing meat without the chemicals and pesticides you risk from non-organic chicken. Enjoy yours with a medley of fresh veggies and a smile on your face

FEELS BAD	FEELS OK	FEELS GOOD

Potato

Fries—an unholy combination of salt and fat. OK, fries can be delicious, but save them for when it really counts, not just an average lunchtime add-on

Baked potato—mayo-based fillings virtually guarantee lethargy, so if you crave this high-GI lunch, then opt for tuna and sweetcorn or chili

Baked sweet potato—fill yours with turkey and avocado. Hey presto, a low-GI lunch with a healthy balance of protein and fat. Add a green salad for an extra feelgood factor

Eggs

Fried egg sandwich—the good you're doing with the egg is undone by the fact it's been fried and squished between slices of high-GI bread

Omelette with cheese and ham—fulfils your protein needs, though eating it with a fresh green salad will make it more satisfying (and less greasy)

Vegetable omelette—often the healthiest choice in a café, but skip the cheese because it's sure to be cooked in more than sufficient fat

Vegetarian

Falafel—how do you make the humble chickpea unhealthy? Deep-fry it

Tofu—a good source of protein, though it soaks up fat like a sponge so watch what you pair it with. Chargrilled vegetables and lemon juice would work beautifully

Lentils—all fifty-plus varieties of lentils are amazing sources of fiber, which is great news for digestive issues. They are also high in folate, which helps your body repair damaged cells. Other pulses like kidney beans, chickpeas and pinto beans are good sources of fiber too, so load up on three-bean salad

Appetizers

Pub apps—chicken goujons, battered calamari, salami, creamy garlic dip and potato wedges. This is processed, deep-fried overload

Packaged apps—sliced ham, stuffed vine leaves, pita bread, cheesy peppers. All OK, but it's easy to overeat if you don't have enough vegetables to fill you up

Fresh vegetable apps—raw rainbow crudités like radishes, cucumber, peppers and carrots give you a satisfying, nutritious crunch, while organic hummus sorts out your protein and healthy fat needs. Usually "reduced-fat" products aren't great, but low-fat hummus is the exception as it substitutes part of the fat for water. Add a seeded pita or some crackers for long-lasting energy

FEELS BAD	FEELS OK	FEELS GOOD

Japanese

White rice sushi with soy sauce, tempura—stop at six pieces because white rice jacks up your insulin. Meanwhile, tempura is unhealthy fried fat you can happily live without. And dousing your meal in soy sauce means too much sodium, which means arugulaing blood pressure

Brown rice sushi with edamame beans—though brown rice is lower GI than white, it is extra sugar that makes it sticky. You don't need soy, as a proper sushi chef prepares the fish exactly as it's meant to be. Edamame beans are OK, too; ask for yours without salt

Sashimi with seaweed salad and pickled ginger—the fish is high in protein and low in fat, while seaweed boasts vitamins A, B, C, E and K and is rich in iodine, selenium and iron. That's what gives it superfood status. Swap tuna for salmon for more heart-healthy omega-3s

Thai

Fried rice, prawn crackers, spring rolls—fatty fried food can worsen heartburn and reflux, which makes for an uncomfortable afternoon

Red or green curry—coconut milk contains lauric acid, which has antiviral and antibacterial properties. Eat yours with stir-fried vegetables rather than rice or noodles

Tom yum soup, papaya salad, grilled chicken satay, prawn and spinach stir-fry—when you cut out the white rice and deep-fried stuff, fresh Thai food is fantastically healthy

Italian

Creamy carbonara or risotto—these contain too many simple carbohydrates, which means you'll feel fatigued all afternoon

Starter portion of pasta or risotto with a side salad—halve the carbs and add a fresh green salad for a better lunch

But if you love spaghetti, have last night's. Reheating cooled pasta makes it resistant to enzymes in your gut that break down carbs, so your meal has a greater proportion of fiber [4]. In other words, it's half as fattening

Mexican

Pork taco with refried beans, cheese and sour cream—pork is the fattiest meat, crispy tacos are fried, refried beans are the unhealthiest way to eat pulses, while cheese and sour cream are extra fat on top of a fattening meal

Beef burrito—use a whole wheat wrap and quality steak for slow-releasing energy and healthy protein. To aid digestion, squeeze lemon over your beef and add black beans for extra fiber

Chicken in a lettuce-wrap burrito—a filling feelgood lunch that won't bloat you and keeps you going until dinnertime. Add guacamole for heart-healthy fat and pinto beans for potassium, which de-puffs your eyes, plus fresh salsa and coriander

HOW TO BUILD THE PERFECT FEELGOOD SALAD

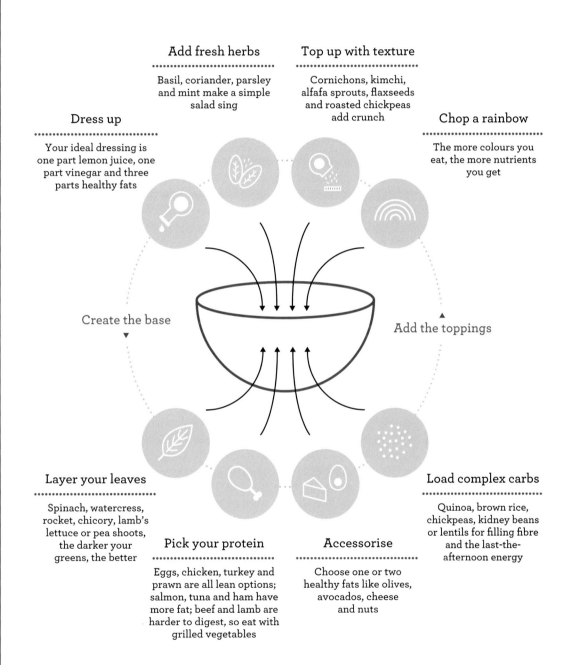

Add fresh herbs
Basil, coriander, parsley and mint make a simple salad sing

Top up with texture
Cornichons, kimchi, alfafa sprouts, flaxseeds and roasted chickpeas add crunch

Dress up
Your ideal dressing is one part lemon juice, one part vinegar and three parts healthy fats

Chop a rainbow
The more colours you eat, the more nutrients you get

Create the base ▼

Add the toppings ▲

Layer your leaves
Spinach, watercress, rocket, chicory, lamb's lettuce or pea shoots, the darker your greens, the better

Pick your protein
Eggs, chicken, turkey and prawn are all lean options; salmon, tuna and ham have more fat; beef and lamb are harder to digest, so eat with grilled vegetables

Accessorise
Choose one or two healthy fats like olives, avocados, cheese and nuts

Load complex carbs
Quinoa, brown rice, chickpeas, kidney beans or lentils for filling fibre and the last-the-afternoon energy

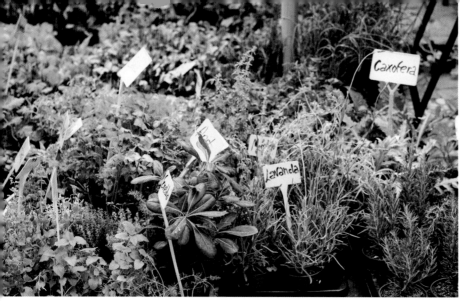

THE FEELGOOD GUIDE TO DINNER

6

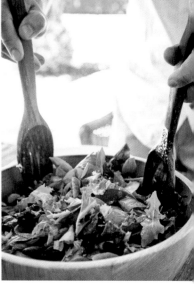

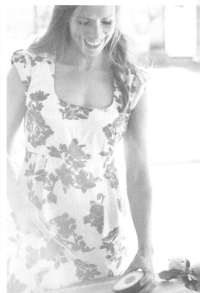

Healthy, home-cooked food doesn't have to be a hassle. Here's how to give your favorite recipes the feelgood factor

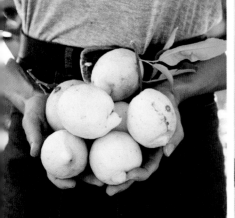

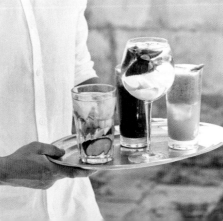

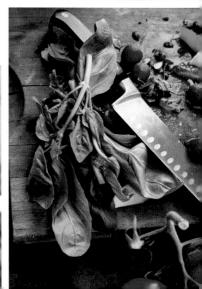

Grandma was right: cooking is the key to making healthy choices [1]. And it's not just eating that nourishes your body. The act of preparing a meal and sharing it with your loved ones will recharge you

Everyone can eat the feelgood way; there's no need to make separate meals for everyone. It's all in the ratios: men typically need more protein, women benefit from having lots more vegetables, while children want a greater balance of complex carbs.

Cook mindfully and you won't pick mindlessly. Focus your senses totally on the now: listen to the knife chopping crisp vegetables, inhale fragrant freshly-ripped coriander, and feel the heat radiating from the pan. When your mind wanders, steer back to the present moment to feel calm, connected and in control.

Portion control is most important at dinner because you're most likely to overeat at the end of the day, and least likely to burn it off. Look at your food diary to remind yourself what you've already eaten today—it's a good indicator of how big a supper you need.

Can't help picking? Just log it in your food diary and be conscious you won't need to eat as much at the table before you're full.

The more flavorsome your food, the more you'll appreciate it. Herbs and spices like ginger, basil and turmeric enhance flavors just as effectively as salt, which is something most of us eat too much of.

An evening bloat will make you feel uncomfortable. If your stomach swells easily, eat grilled, stir-fried and steamed vegetables over raw ones, and choose white meat instead of red as it can digest three times faster. Squeeze lemon over your dinner: the juice tenderizes the meat and begins breaking down the proteins. Lemon helps bring out the flavor of your food, too.

Take at least 15 minutes to cook a delicious, nutritious, satisfying dinner instead of making do with whatever you can grab instantly

THE 5 COMMANDMENTS OF COOKING FOR 1

Eating solo can get you into a cycle of unhealthy habits like overeating and relying on convenience food. But it doesn't have to be that way

1 Honour thyself

When you cook just for yourself, you don't have to compromise to please someone else. Rustle up feelgood food that makes your mouth water and spice it to suit you.

2 Thou shalt feel good

None of us are strangers to the antisocial dinner. You know: a box of cereal, a whole rice pudding, a giant bag of chips. Filling yourself with food that has no physiological benefit has no psychological benefit either. Before you tuck in, ask yourself, "Will this really make me feel good?" If the answer is yes, go right ahead. If it's no, then make yourself a feelgood dinner (see the grid on the next page) and don't keep foods that make you feel bad in the house.

3 Thou shalt make life easy

Don't see the point of cooking for one? Cook several portions and box them up straight away for lunch tomorrow or stash in the freezer for future zero-effort dinners.

4 Thou shalt not overeat

Dining solo puts you in the fortunate position of being able to completely connect with your food without distractions from other people, so you're more aware when you're full. Sit at the table and chew each bite carefully, feeling the tastes and textures in your mouth. You'll feel physically and mentally satisfied, so won't accidentally overeat. When you're done, get up from the table so you don't idly pick at leftovers.

5 Thou shalt not forget simple options

Opening a supermarket salad bowl is as quick and easy as opening a box of cereal, but way better for you. When you're stressed out and in danger of sliding down the antisocial eating shute, add arugula to your salad. The peppery green leaf is a good source of folates, which help even out mood swings. Here's the science: folates lower levels of an amino acid called homocysteine. High levels of homocysteine interfere with the flow of nutrients to the brain, making you prone to highs and lows.

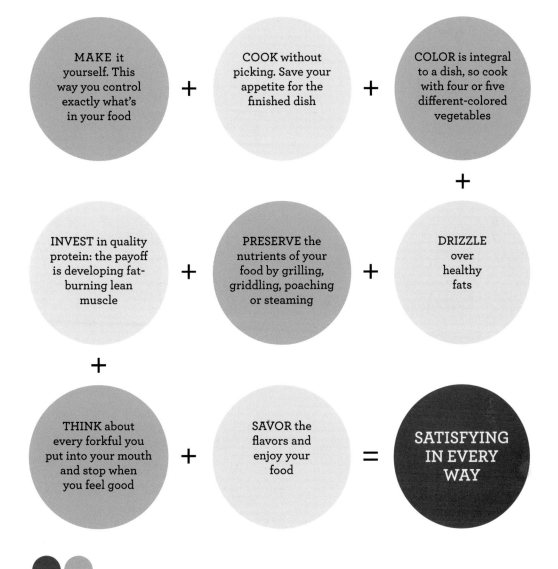

MAKE it yourself. This way you control exactly what's in your food

+

COOK without picking. Save your appetite for the finished dish

+

COLOR is integral to a dish, so cook with four or five different-colored vegetables

+

INVEST in quality protein: the payoff is developing fat-burning lean muscle

+

PRESERVE the nutrients of your food by grilling, griddling, poaching or steaming

+

DRIZZLE over healthy fats

+

THINK about every forkful you put into your mouth and stop when you feel good

+

SAVOR the flavors and enjoy your food

=

SATISFYING IN EVERY WAY

Want more even though you're not hungry?
Try thinking of your favorite activity—maybe playing with a dog or laughing with your best friend. Simple visualisations can lessen cravings [2].

INSPIRATION FOR 20 FEELGOOD DINNERS

FEELS BAD	FEELS OK	FEELS GOOD

Burger and fries

Non-organic meat may contain pesticides and chemicals and is usually bulked out with cheap rusk. Put in a white bun with processed cheese, add fries and ketchup and you have a high-calorie dinner that makes you feel tired afterwards

Buy free-range meat and put in a whole wheat bun for a cleaner burger. Serve with sweet potato fries and a fresh side salad

Make your burger with organic ground meat and eat it on an open-faced whole wheat bun to halve the carbs. Bake sweet potato wedges and make a big salad with avocado, tomatoes, arugula, watercress and radishes. All that fiber helps you digest the red meat

Chilli con carne

Heaps of factory-farmed meat, only a handful of kidney beans and a mountain of white rice is an unhealthy balance. The meat is tasteless, so you're compelled to bury it under a greasy mound of cheese. To make this chili worse, white rice is high GI, which sets your blood sugar up for a crash

Use free-range meat, plenty of kidney beans and only a little whole grain rice—the healthiest way to add carbohydrates is to cook with extra vegetables. Onion, tomato and peppers are all a must. Include fresh chilies too: they contain capsaicin, which is clinically proven to speed up weight loss [3]. A small handful of cheddar on top makes this chili extra satisfying

Feelgood chili is composed of equal parts organic meat, beans and vegetables. Use a variety for extra benefits: pinto, kidney and black beans all taste good. Add plenty of veggies like onion, leek, mushroom, eggplant and yellow pepper for filling complex carbs and fiber. Serve your chili on a bed of cauliflower rice (see page 92 for your how-to). On top, add extra slices of fresh chilies to boost your metabolism, then grate over a little organic Parmesan—a small pinch gives a big flavor and just ⅛ cup delivers 15% of your daily calcium

Fish and chips

Battered fish and chips with tinned mushy peas and lots of ketchup = a greasy cocktail of chemicals, trans-fats and sugar. Your body doesn't know how to process these, so you store the toxins in your fat cells

Cut down on trans-fats and refined carbs by pan-frying your cod and eating it with a baked potato, buttery peas and a dollop of tartar sauce

Fish and chips is easily transformed into a feelgood meal. Bake your cod in a foil parcel with plenty of lemon. Roast sweet potato wedges with chunky carrots, beetroot and red pepper, then add a fresh pea purée for a nutritious, mood-boosting rainbow of vegetables

FEELS BAD	FEELS OK	FEELS GOOD

Frittata

Putting more potato than eggs into your frittata means too much carbohydrate and not enough protein, especially when you use high-GI white potatoes and there's no salad in sight

It's OK to make your frittata with half free-range eggs and half new potatoes, but keep the skins on your potatoes as these are loaded with fiber. Do your body a favor and toss a salad on the side, too

Cook the ultimate feelgood frittata with organic free-range eggs, sweet potato, kale, Swiss chard, onion and peas, then serve on a bed of watercress with a fresh tomato salsa

Indian chicken tikka

Drop pan-fried, factory-farmed chicken into a creamy masala sauce and put it on a bed of white rice, and you have a curry that makes you feel sluggish for hours afterwards. Naan bread, poppadoms and sticky mango chutney jack up your insulin even more and make the after-dinner slump feel even worse

Forget masala; tikka is the healthiest, yummiest part. Marinate chunks of chicken from your local butcher in grated ginger, garlic, yogurt, lime juice, fresh coriander, turmeric, chili, garam masala and paprika, and use the same mixture to blend for the sauce. Mix diced red onion and peas into your whole grain rice to up the vegetable count

To make this curry feel really good, buy organic chicken and chargrill it instead of frying. Simply thread your marinated chicken chunks onto skewers and balance them across a baking tray in your oven for 30 minutes. Eat your chicken with an Indian salad of cucumber, tomatoes, chili and onion, and serve dahl instead of rice—red lentils are a great low-fat source of plant protein and fiber

Lamb steak

Breast, the belly area of lamb, is the fattiest cut. And it's even fattier when you fry it. Avoid honey-glazed carrots as they're basically covered in sugar. Instant gravy cubes or powders are full of nasty preservatives

Upgrade your lamb by buying free-range and grilling it. Add three vegetables—try kale, carrots and purple broccoli. Make your own gravy with the meat juices, some vegetable water and whole wheat flour

Loin, shank and leg are the leanest cuts of lamb. Buy organic, cover it in rosemary and griddle it so the fat drains away. Eat with kale, Chinese cabbage, purple broccoli, carrots and mushrooms, then drizzle with a home-made jus

Moussaka

When topped with a gloopy, shop-bought béchamel sauce, filled with poor-quality ground lamb and fried, breadcrumbed eggplant, the result makes you feel lethargic

Moussaka topped with grated cheese instead of white sauce, then filled with lamb from your local butcher and pan-fried strips of eggplant. A hearty yet wholesome dinner

Sprinkle your moussaka with organic Parmesan cheese, grill your eggplant so it's less fatty, and fill it with organic 100% grass-fed lamb. This meat has 25% more omega-3s than grain-fed lamb [4]. Add plenty of rosemary, too

FEELS BAD	FEELS OK	FEELS GOOD

Mackerel skewers

A meager portion of mackerel with white rice is pretty boring and doesn't feel substantial enough to satisfy your hunger, either	Mackerel is often shunned in favor of salmon, yet it has twice the amount of heart-healthy, anti-inflammatory omega-3 fatty acids as the popular pink fish. Try pan-fried mackerel with low-sodium teriyaki sauce, whole grain rice and a fresh green side salad	Make mackerel feel really good by eating it ceviche-style. All you need is fresh fish, lime juice and cucumber. The juice of one lime per fish should do. Chop and mix these ingredients. Five minutes later, the fish is "cooked" in the acidity of the citrus. Though lime is acid itself, it has a feelgood alkalining effect on the body. Serve your ceviche skewers on a bed of grilled vegetables and drizzle with olive oil for an extra dose of healthy fats

Mussels

Mussels are low in calories— but not when cooked in wine and double cream, or when you soak up the sauce with fries or sugary white bread	Make your marinière sauce with crème frâiche instead of double cream and add tarragon to bring out the flavor. Serve with whole wheat bread for slow-releasing energy	Steam your mussels in a lemony tomato broth and serve with dark rye bread for maximum feelgood benefits. Mussels are a great source of brain-enhancing fats and energising iron and zinc, which support your immune system

Risotto

White rice, smoked supermarket bacon, non-organic cream and a lump of processed, sawdusty Parmesan on top … you're not going to feel great eating this	Risotto is better made with whole grain rice and plenty of vegetables: try asparagus, peas and spring onions. Ask your butcher for unsmoked lardons as these deliver a salty, robust flavor with less chemicals. Use ricotta instead of cream— it gives you extra protein and one serving provides half of your daily recommended calcium intake, which balances out the fact you've added extra fat	Primavera is the healthiest risotto recipe—cook yours with less whole grain rice and more feelgood ingredients like broad beans, asparagus, peas, spring onions, collard greens and lemon zest. Broad beans are the key ingredient: they're a good plant source of protein and fiber and high in folate and B-vitamins, which we use in nerve and blood cell development, for cognitive function and energy. For a creamy taste with extra protein, stir a beaten egg into your risotto in the last few minutes on the stove. Pecorino cheese is full of flavor, so you don't need a handful; just a sprinkle on top will do the business

FEELS BAD	FEELS OK	FEELS GOOD

Salmon and new potatoes

Buy farmed salmon, cover it in cheesy breadcrumbs, fry it, add a massive pile of new potatoes, smother it in creamy sauce and you have a high-carb, high-fat fish dish. Farmed salmon is worryingly high in PCBs, an industrial chemical waste [5]

Pan-frying organic salmon is OK, especially when you drizzle it with the butter you fried it in instead of adding a cream sauce. Eat with new potatoes, steamed broccoli and mushrooms

Bake your wild-caught salmon in a foil parcel with lemon, fresh herbs and salt to bring out its flavor and make this fish even more satisfying. Serve with new potatoes and four other vegetables that are in season now—nutrients are at their peak when eaten in season

Spaghetti carbonara

White pasta is high GI so it's hard not to overeat carbonara this way. White garlic bread just piles up the problem. Factory-farmed eggs, inorganic double cream, cheese and smoked bacon mean more toxic animal pesticides and antibiotics stored in your fat cells

Spaghetti carbonara made with wholewheat pasta, free-range eggs, crème fraîche, free-range bacon and locally produced cheese. Make your own garlic bread with a whole wheat baguette and use butter instead of margarine

Corn pasta, organic free-range eggs and organic unsmoked bacon is the healthiest way to enjoy carbonara. You don't need actual cream: cheese alone makes the dish taste creamy. If pasta is a non-negotiable want for you, eat it al dente—cooked this way spaghetti has a lower GI [7]. The carbs are released into your bloodstream more slowly, so you feel satisfied for longer. Balance the acidic bacon out by filling half your plate with watercress, arugula and spinach, dressed with lemon

Shepherd's pie

Low-quality supermarket ground meat, refined white potato on top and sugary processed ketchup splattered everywhere, this shepherd's pie won't satisfy you for long

Ground lamb or beef from your local butcher cooked with onions, carrots and celery, plus mashed sweet potato for the crust, makes you feel better. The extra veggies provide fiber that helps digest meat faster so it doesn't sit heavily in your stomach

Shepherd's pie made with organic ground lamb or beef, carrots, celery, skin-on mashed sweet potato and a peppery salad bursting with arugula, watercress, radishes, cucumber and tomato. Hey presto: a perfect balance of quality protein, complex carbs, fiber and nutritious vegetables

FEELS BAD	FEELS OK	FEELS GOOD

Squid

Calamari makes you feel bad because deep-frying means adding unhealthy trans-fats and tripling the calorie count	Squid is a good source of lean protein, omega-3, copper, zinc, B-vitamins and iodine, which are vital for muscle growth, forming healthy red blood cells and strengthening your immune system. Breadcrumb and pan-fry the squid yourself	The healthiest way to eat squid is to grill it with butter and lemon, then serve on a big bed of colorful vegetable ratatouille. Butternut squash, broccoli, courgettes, red and orange peppers and samphire all go beautifully with squid

Steak and fries

A pan-fried T-bone is one of the fattiest ways to eat steak, and fries are high in unhealthy trans-fats, sodium and refined carbohydrates. It's worth repeating that eating mass-produced, inorganic meat means you're eating animal pesticides, too	Ask your local butcher for a bavette—a large flat cut of steak that's better value than supermarket meat and, because it's farmed locally, it's more nutritious, too. Griddle it and eat with oven-baked potato wedges, carrots and broccoli	Sirloin is the leanest cut of beef. Grill an organic, grass-fed steak and oven-cook sweet potato wedges. Serve with a side of steamed asparagus, broccoli, mushrooms and kale and horseradish: alkaline foods that balance out the natural acidity of the meat

Tagine

Cooking with processed, pesticide-infused meat won't delight your taste buds, or indeed any part of your body. Couscous and dried fruit are both high-GI, so eating a mountain of the stuff has the same effect as consuming a white baguette: your blood sugar will spike and crash	One of the best things about tagine is that it makes a feast from inexpensive cuts—ask your butcher for lamb neck or beef shin. After a few hours in a warm oven, your meat will fall apart beautifully. Throw in butternut squash, onion and tomato to make it filling, and go easy on sugary dried fruit	When you use equal quantities of quality meat and vegetables, this is a real feelgood meal. Butternut squash, onion, tomato, aubergine and green pepper all work brilliantly. Replace couscous with quinoa—this complex carb delivers protein, too. Squeeze lemon over a green salad for extra freshness

Thai prawn stir-fry

Factory-farmed prawns are packed with toxins. Shop-bought curry sauce is full of preservatives and unhealthy fat. Instant noodles are highly processed and full of sodium, which is linked to cardiovascular disease	It's OK to use Thai curry paste from a jar, but add an extra pinch of turmeric as this spice is unusually high in disease-fighting anti-inflammatories [8]. Throw in your own fresh green beans, spring onions and beansprouts, too. Rice noodles are gluten-free, which means they're less likely to bloat you	Buy prawns from your fishmonger for the freshest local catch. No noodles required: stir-fry your prawns in coconut oil with Thai basil, lime juice, garlic, ginger, spring onions, beansprouts, Chinese cabbage and green beans for maximum taste and minimum sugar

FEELS BAD	FEELS OK	FEELS GOOD

Turkey stir-fry

Cooking with factory-farmed turkey, a heap of wheat noodles and gloopy, MSG-laden sauce from a jar means stuffing your stomach with a lot of foreign chemicals

Turkey thighs are the best value free-range white meat. If you have to have noodles, buy the glass rice variety as they're naturally gluten-free so less likely to make you feel bloated and tired. Throw three different vegetables into your stir-fry: try onion, courgette and colorful peppers to add antioxidants

Make this meal feel good by stir-frying organic turkey with chilies, ginger, onion, garlic, mushrooms, courgette, yellow pepper, Brussels sprouts and kale. Try courgette noodles to fill you up with the best-quality complex carbs. Top with fresh coriander and use turkey breast as it is leaner than thigh meat

Vegetable stir-fry

Many meat substitutes made from textured vegetable protein (TVP) are chemically manipulated and sodden with pesticides. Scour the food label to see exactly what it contains: a huge ingredients list is usually a bad sign. Watch out for high sodium content, too, especially if you're tempted by the convenience of instant noodles and processed package sauce

Tofu, or soya bean curd, is a good plant-based source of amino acids, iron and calcium. It's fairly healthy paired with a fresh supermarket sauce and stir-fried. Some vegetables can be a stealthy source of protein, so be generous with peas, spinach and Brussels sprouts

Go one better with tempeh. Also made from soya beans, the tempeh fermentation process and its retention of the whole bean mean that it packs more protein, dietary fiber and vitamins than tofu. Make your sauce with plenty of lemon, herbs, ginger and garlic. Get more protein power from your veggies and make them colorful for extra feelgood factor: try purple-sprouting broccoli and sweetcorn as well as your peas, Chinese cabbage and Swiss chard. Serve with cashews and fresh herbs for extra flavor

OK. Maybe green vegetables aren't your thing...

You know nutritional powerhouses like kale, Chinese cabbage, watercress, arugula, Swiss chard, broccoli, Brussels sprouts and collard greens are exceptionally good for you. You know these great greens can give you glowing skin, skim off a spare tyre, energize every single cell in your body and even reduce your risk of chronic diseases like cancer[10]. Whatever. You just can't stand them. So here's your three-step rehab program:

1 Dress up your greens:
Accessorize your vegetable nemesis with a taste you do like. Stir-fry Brussels sprouts with unsmoked pancetta, cook broccoli with soy sauce, grate Parmesan over kale. Several meals later, your brain forms a positive association with both tastes. In a few weeks, you'll discover you like the greens au naturel, too.

2 Put greens on the right side of your plate:
We usually fork from that side first, so you'll eat more vegetables without having to try too hard [11].

3 Get out of the kitchen:
If you can't stand the smell of boiled cabbage, eat it in a different room. It may just be the odour you don't like. Your sense of smell is weakest in the evening, so you could find vegetables surprisingly delicious with dinner.

More plate pain = less weight gain.

The labour-intensive act of shelling prawns, scooping mussels from their shell or forking up a multi-textured salad means you have to eat more mindfully.

Love mayo but want to stay healthy? Mix Greek yogurt with fresh basil or rosemary. The herbs have anti-inflammatory compounds and yogurt delivers immune-boosting probiotics.

Would you like...

... a glass of wine?

That's cool; wine's sugar is absorbed slower when you pair Pinot Noir with your meal. The occasional glass of red is good for your heart [12] and also helps control cholesterol [13]. What's more, wine can help ward off food poisoning [14].

... some cheese?

Cheese won't give you nightmares. Enjoy a matchbox-sized portion of your favorite flavor, and savor it. Eating a whole cheese plate is like mainlining a massive family-sized cake, especially if it comes with crackers, chutney and grapes.

... a sweet treat?

Dessert is a habit, not a real nutritional need. If you'd like to be slimmer but you can't help pining for pudding, try adding sweet tastes to your meal to stop the craving before it starts. Add sautéed onions to stir-fries, sprinkle cinnamon on mashed sweet potatos or chop pears into salad. Still want dessert? Try the healthy sweet treats on page 117.

Still want more?

If you can't take the temptation, stay out of the kitchen. Even better, get some fresh air: walking for 15 minutes seriously reduces cravings [15]. The beauty of a craving is that once your mind is off it, the intensity vanishes.

Keep these home-cooked meals in the freezer

Enjoy taking time to batch-cook one or two meals every week—it's an investment in your body

Chilli, both vegetarian and beef-based

Lasagne made with grilled peppers and courgettes instead of pasta

Stews like lentil and sweet potato or beef stroganoff

Moussaka with a cheesy, eggy topping

Cottage or shepherd's pie with mashed sweet potatos

Fish pie with soft-boiled eggs inside and mashed sweet potatos on top

Ratatouille made with chunky vegetables

Dahl made with lentils, mushrooms and peas

Curry: as well as the classic chicken, try butternut squash and eggplant

Fish cakes with a crunchy almond coating

Tagine with beef, chicken, or lamb and hearty root vegetables

Meatballs: try lamb and rosemary

Chicken and bean enchiladas

Fish or meat skewers: freeze after marinating

All soups freeze well

5–6pm

If you eat early to fit around your kids' schedule, neither be fooled into fobbing yourself off with a child's portion—thus eating too little—or into picking at your kids' leftovers and eating too much. Seal any food worth keeping into airtight boxes and scrape everything else into the bin.

If you get hungry later in the evening, have a light snack that's easy on your stomach. Sliced apple with cheese or homemade banana ice cream (the easy-peasy recipe is on page 117) will do nicely. You don't need another dinner—you've already eaten! So if that doesn't satisfy your hunger, it's not food you're hungry for, it's rest. Get an early night.

7–8pm

This is the ideal time to eat, as it gives you enough time to cook, sit down to enjoy your meal, then 3 hours to relax and digest before you go to sleep.

9–10pm

When you've been out with friends, to the gym after work or get stuck late in the office, eating late is unavoidable. Choose easily digestible foods like eggs over red meat, which can sit heavily in your stomach. If you're still digesting while you sleep, your body can't carry out all of its usual night-time repairs as well. Take the load off your stomach by eating a smaller portion.

It's tempting to gorge on comfort foods when you're tired. However, eating sugar and refined carbs late in the evening will jack up your insulin and the following crash may wake you up in the middle of the night. That's the last thing you need when you're already tired. Instead of eating a carb-heavy meal that your body doesn't have time to burn off, your best plan is to eat a light meal—an omelette is ideal—then go to bed.

Go-go-gadget arms

When you have time, cook without using a food processor. Beating eggs, chopping vegetables and stirring the pan all help tone your arms.

UPGRADE YOUR EVENING EATING HABITS
It's not just what you munch, it's the way that you crunch it

STOP THIS	DO THIS
Watching TV. When you're gripped by a great program, you can eat up to 44% more food without realising [16]. Research also shows that you're much more likely to overeat while watching a cookery show	Eating at the table improves digestion because you eat slower and when you're not distracted, you appreciate your food more. People who eat their meals at a table consume fewer calories at their next meal [17]
Picking at your children's dinner, then eating an adult supper later too means you end up eating two dinners	If you want to eat with your children, cook extra vegetables and have a small plate of them. Later, at supper, serve yourself a smaller portion than your partner. Effectively, you're taking one meal and dividing it in two
Bright light makes you stressed so you eat too much too fast. Think about the lighting in fast food restaurants—it's designed that way so you won't pay close attention to what you eat and so you'll cram it down in a hurry	Eat by candlelight. The mellow mood helps you unwind, which slows the speed you eat and allows your mind to sync with your stomach, so you stop eating when you're full [18]. Can't see what you're eating in candlelight? Use a side lamp or switch to a 13-watt bulb
Mindless eating while cooking means you end up eating double the volume	Sip water as you cook. When you sit down to eat you'll appreciate your food more, and because you won't be dehydrated, you can gauge your hunger better. It's best to drink before a meal, not during it, because water can dilute your digestive enzymes

STOP THIS

Gorging on comfort foods high in sugar, refined carbs and unhealthy fats means you're setting yourself up to overeat, have stomach pain, then feel hungry all over again. Doing this regularly is a sure-fire formula for misery and weight gain

Dishing up seconds, thirds and an extra spoonful too…

Eating another spoonful from the pan, rummaging in the fridge for snacks and scavenging in your kitchen cupboards. So you're pretty much eating the whole evening long

DO THIS

Eating a balanced dinner with plenty of vegetables, a portion of lean protein, some healthy fats and complex carbohydrates makes you feel satisfied, calm and it sets your body up for a great night's sleep

Dish up at the kitchen counter instead of at the table so that the pan isn't in easy reach. If you've cooked more than one portion, pack the extras away immediately so you're not tempted to overeat

When your meal is over, get up from the table and put the food away so you're not tempted to pick at it. Make yourself a cup of peppermint tea to help your digestion and mark the end of your meal

When you're eating out, going to a dinner party or throwing one yourself, do it in a way that makes you feel good. See page 103 for your how-to.

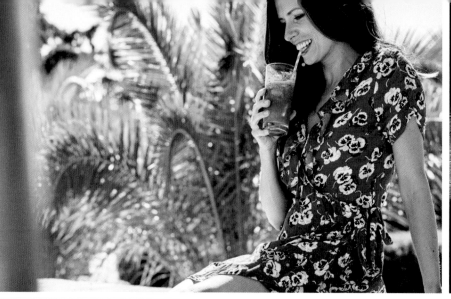

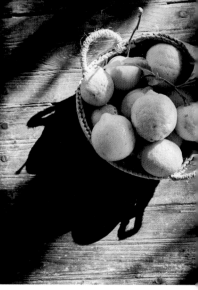

WILLPOWER, CRAVINGS, SNACKS AND YOU 7

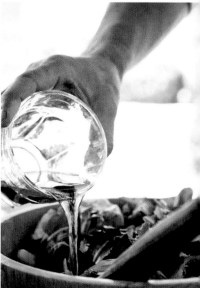

So, you know what foods make you feel good, and what's worth avoiding. How do you actually make it happen? By tapping into your emotional intelligence

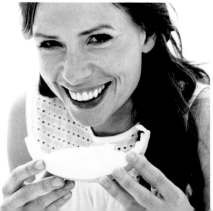

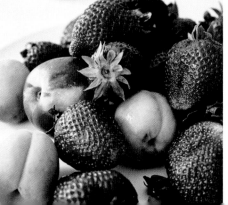

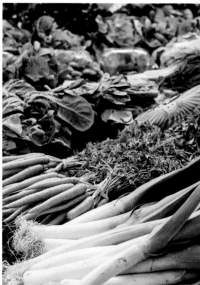

Couldn't you just kill for a cookie right now? We've all been there, done that and looked at the empty package wondering what just happened. Having cravings doesn't make you weak, it makes you human. It makes you normal: a whopping 97% of women and 68% of men experience episodes of food cravings [1]

Just because you have the occasional desperate urge to steal candy from the nearest baby doesn't mean you have to give in if doing so makes you feel bad. Because, believe it or not, you have plenty of willpower. Honestly, you do. It's all in there, even if it's buried deep. And willpower is like a muscle: the more you use it, the stronger it gets.

How can you pump up yours? Glad you asked. The more you're aware of how your mood is affected by what you eat, the more you'll understand how to make positive, healthy changes. When you notice you're repeating a bad habit, you can consciously make a smarter choice—one that makes you feel good. As you develop a deeper understanding of your body's relationship with food, you'll realize your inner strength. This chapter will guide you.

The link between sugar and aging.

Sugar cells bind to elastin and collagen proteins—the ingredients that give your skin a youthful bounce—and make them unable to repair. So the higher your blood sugar, the faster your skin will wrinkle. Having elevated blood sugar also makes your mood spike and crash. The lows sap your energy, so you feel old. This completes the sweet triple threat: too much sugar ages your liver, so you can't process insulin efficiently, which means gaining weight— or what your mother might call a "middle-aged spread'.

Walking for 15 minutes is the best way to overcome unhealthy cravings—it's 1% of your day well spent

Do you really need a snack right now?

When you eat three good meals, snacks aren't a necessary part of your day. Use this guide to read your internal body language, so you know when and how to check in with your body. Because if hunger isn't the problem, eating isn't the answer

	It's less than 2 hours since you last ate	It's an hour until lunch or dinner	It's 15 minutes until your next meal
HEAD	Cast your mind back to your last meal. Even 3 hours after eating, thinking about what you consumed earlier in the day cuts down your calorie intake and curbs your urge to snack [2]	Are you bored or stressed? Distract yourself from thinking about food with a change of scenery. A 15-minute walk will relax your body and take your mind off food for at least 25 minutes [3]	Is your mind foggy? You need to eat. Prepare food that boosts your brainpower. Salmon is rich in brain-nourishing omega-3s and broccoli is a great source of vitamin K, which is proven to enhance brain function. Start stir-frying
HEART	Has your hunger come on suddenly? You're emotionally hungry: physical hunger occurs gradually [4]. Feed your feelings by phoning a friend—it's far more effective than comfort food	Do you need a pick-me-up? Boost your mood with sunlight or gentle exercise—fresh air, vitamin D from the sun and increased oxygen flow from exercise all increase serotonin, the happy hormone, better than food can	Focus on exactly what you'd like to eat and start preparing your meal. Anticipation makes any food from carrot sticks to chocolate cake taste better and feel more emotionally satisfying [5]
STOMACH	Actually, do you still feel a little heavy from your last meal? Peppermint tea will soothe that discomfort—eating now will make you feel worse	Thirst is often mistaken for hunger, so have a glass of water. Drink sparkling or lemon-infused water to placate your taste buds as well as your stomach	Has your hunger gradually increased since you last checked in with your body? Then it's true hunger: you need to bring dinner forward a little

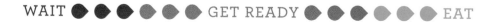

WAIT ⬤ ⬤ ⬤ ⬤ ⬤ ⬤ GET READY ⬤ ⬤ ⬤ ⬤ ⬤ ⬤ EAT

FIVE WAYS TO WAKE UP YOUR WILLPOWER
Because a firm body starts with having a firm mind

1 Eat. Eating a more plant-based, less processed diet not only gives your body a steady supply of energy, but eating clean, nutritious food makes that energy more available to your brain, which can strengthen your willpower [6]. More nuts, less chicken nuggets.

2 Plan. Being busy screws with your self-control. Planning puts willpower back in the game, so even when you're rushed, you can make effortlessly good food choices. Keep a stash of hard-boiled eggs in the fridge to keep you going when you've got more than 4 hours between meals. This feelgood snack contains amino acids, which dilate blood vessels so oxygen flows more easily and you'll find it easier to tick off your to-do list on a busy day. Almonds are a great snack to stash in your handbag as they are high in a heart-healthy fat called oleic acid that can boost memory [7].

3 Be subtle. Change "I can't" to "I don't". Why? "I can't eat chips," means "I'm not allowed to eat chips," and forbidden foods are impossibly desirable. Give your willpower a fighting chance by saying, "I don't eat chips'. Because you're actually saying, "I prefer not to eat chips; they don't make me feel good'. The difference is subtle, but empowering.

4 Rebrand. If you describe yourself as a latte lover or a fried chicken fiend, people will constantly push those temptations in front of you. They think they're doing you a favor. Do yourself a favor and rebrand. Tell friends you're obsessed with green juice, because you can practically feel those antioxidants replenishing your body. When you're choosing where to go for dinner, tell your partner you've got a thing about grass-fed steak. When you talk the talk, it naturally follows that you walk the walk.

5 Breathe. Learning how to manage your stress better, even if it's just taking a few deep breaths when you feel tempted, is one of the most important things you can do to improve your self-control [8]. So as you stare at a counter full of glazed pastries, take a few deep breaths to gather your willpower and order a feelgood fix instead. Black coffee sweetened with a dash of cinnamon or a piece of fresh fruit with some raw nuts will see you right.

What kind of emotional eater are you?
Take this quiz to stop being sabotaged by bad habits and put feeling good into practice

From birthday cake to Christmas turkey or the cup of tea you make for a friend, food is intrinsically linked with our emotions. We eat when we're busy, bored, happy, sad and every shade of grey between.

Feeding our feelings, not our stomachs, is a huge issue. Emotional eating is the single biggest reason for weight gain and fatigue—it's estimated that 75% of what we eat is governed by our emotions [9]. That means no matter how often you exercise or how sensible you try to be with your food choices the rest of the time, emotional eating will sabotage your feelgood goal. If you don't get a grip on emotional eating, you will put on weight, be tired and feel powerless around food. Yes, it's tricky to resist a bag of chips after an exhausting day, but it's not as difficult as losing the weight gained from overindulging all the time. Let's sort this out.

So how do we stop emotional eating? Upping our emotional intelligence—the ability to perceive, control and evaluate our emotions—helps us make smarter decisions about what we put in our mouths [10].

Take this quiz to ID those thoughts that sabotage your healthy intentions, and you will discover how to overcome emotional eating. Tick all of the statements that apply, then read on to reveal your emotional eating personality.

Junk food isn't much of a reward if it makes you feel bad, is it?

- [ ] You've been exercising iron willpower all day, then you get home and binge

- [x] **You often finish off what's left in the saucepan so it doesn't go to waste**

- [ ] Your boss has baked cupcakes. You'd be rude to refuse

- [ ] Self-consciousness stops you overeating around people, but alone, you lose it

- [ ] At a dinner party, the host offers seconds and you feel obliged to have more, though you're already full

- [x] **There's only one solution to a fight with your sister: ice cream**

- [x] **You frequently eat food you don't particularly like, just because it's there**

- [x] Overeating makes you stress about the thought of putting on weight

- [ ] You hide the pile of sweet wrappers in the bin, like nothing ever happened

- [ ] Your friends can always rely on you to go out when they want to have fun

- [x] **When you're busy at work, you keep treats on standby in your drawer**

- [x] **Before your appetizer arrives, you accidentally fill up on the bread basket**

- [ ] By yourself in the kitchen, you raid the fridge

- [ ] A tray of sausage rolls is passed round the party. You aren't hungry, but it would be rude to refuse

- [x] **You barely noticed emptying that package of sweets as you drove home**

- [ ] **Your commute took twice as long as it should, so you deserve a big dinner**

It's normal to be a mix of eating personalities, so read all the advice that applies

Mostly red: you're a stress-eater

You snack to cope with everyday stress like a hellish commute and when disaster strikes, you launch into a serious feeding frenzy. Food is your go-to emotional crutch. But it's a negative spiral because when you inevitably gain weight, overeating becomes a stressor in itself.

I can't get away from my desk, I'm too busy

I'd be more productive if I took a break and ate brain food— and I'd stop overeating, too

I deserve a giant pizza, I've had a really manic day

I'm tired because I've got a post-sugar slump. I'll balance my energy with fish and sweet potatos for dinner, then have an early night

Dismiss sabotaging stress-eating thoughts and listen to your body

OVERCOME STRESS EATING

Saying "just relax" is pointless: stress-eaters manage stress by taking action. Exercise is the best method to distract you from your racing mind, and it has the bonus of regulating your appetite, increasing the flow of energising oxygen and releasing endorphins, the stress-diffusing hormone. If you can't put your trainers on right now, maybe dance to the radio, take a walk or discreetly stretch at your desk by clasping your palms behind your back.

Break the stress-eating habit by planning what you want to eat at least a day in advance—a regular pattern is proven to help maintain a healthy weight [11]. So get groceries delivered, batch-cook or pick up feelgood convenience foods like a salad bowl with rotisserie chicken from the supermarket—remind yourself of the best grab-and-go lunches on page 52. During exceptionally busy times, treat yourself to a meal delivery service.

What to eat? Your brain is 60% fat, so essential fatty acids are, yes, essential for better brain function [12]. Salmon, avocado, eggs, nuts, olive oil and coconut oil are all great feelgood choices. Pair them with complex carbs like sweet potato, brown rice and quinoa for energy to last until your next meal.

Onto the "when'. If you're a heart surgeon elbow deep in a patient, then you can't stop what you're doing to eat lunch. Everyone else can escape their desk for 15 minutes. Not only does that break make you more productive (you could even leave the office on time tonight, imagine!) but that time spent focusing on your food makes a simple meal more satisfying. Paying attention to the colors, textures and tastes of your food means you'll eat less, yet stay fuller—and happier—for longer. Goodbye, energy-sapping afternoon snacks.

Now, the "how'. As a busy eater, you know all about eating in a hurry. Change your ways by choosing food you can't eat in two gulps. Use utensils. Salads are great because they contain lots of different textures and protein is also good because you have to chew it thoroughly. If you're still bothered by bloating and other digestive discomforts, squeeze lemon on meat to help break it down and take a digestive enzyme supplement afterwards.

FOOD DIARY TIP FOR STRESS EATERS

As well as noting your mood before and after stress eating, observe when you do it. If a regular Monday meeting is like a siren call to snack, plan to take a walk or do an easy workout (see page 134) afterwards instead.

Blame your gut for junk food cravings

Bad bacteria in your gut could be responsible for certain cravings [13]. This unhealthy bacteria sends out signals to the body, encouraging you to consume the sugar and fat that it thrives on. Honestly, it's enough to put you right off your kebab. Feed the healthy bacteria in your gut with probiotics like sauerkraut to sort it out.

Mostly blue: you're a people pleaser

You eat "to be polite" rather than choosing what's right for you. Whether it's Sunday lunch with your family, cookies in the office or having seconds because your friend insists she'll feel like a greedy pig if you don't have some too, you're forced into eating food that makes you feel bad because you don't want to make a fuss.

It would be rude to refuse

Saying "no thank you" isn't rude—but it is rude of others to force food on me

I'm stuffed, but I don't want to seem like a killjoy

It's OK to say I ate earlier if I'm not hungry

Dismiss sabotaging people-pleasing ideas and listen to your body

OVERCOME EATING TO PLEASE OTHERS

For some people, providing food is the way they show love and affection. Let them know you appreciate them with a diplomatic, "No thank you, I ate earlier', if you're not hungry. Practise saying it with conviction so the words come out effortlessly and a food-pusher doesn't bulldoze you into submission.

Home-made food is harder to refuse because of the time, care and attention that has gone in to making it. But if you know eating all of that sugary icing will make your stomach balloon uncomfortably, then don't eat it. Compliment the cook: "Your cupcakes look delicious, what's your recipe?" This shifts the focus from eating to learning how to make it.

A friend is not going to have a problem with your answer. It's worth bearing in mind that some people love baking, but don't like to eat what they make. So if they don't want to, you shouldn't feel obliged either! People's comments can also be a reflection of their own food issues. Reassure them by saying, "Why don't you have a slice? Enjoy!" This also helps take the focus off you.

There's no need to become a recluse—being with family and friends is one of life's best mood-boosters. So focus on spending quality time with your loved ones instead of using those get-togethers as an excuse to eat. Instead of always eating and drinking to excess, do an exercise class with your friends, get your nails done together, go for a bike ride or simply meet for a coffee without getting a slice of carrot cake too. Chances are your friends are experiencing exactly the same "I wish fun times didn't make me feel bad" frustration as you, and they will welcome your healthier habits.

FOOD DIARY TIP FOR PEOPLE PLEASERS

Observe where you eat and who you eat with. If there's a particular venue where you always feel overstuffed, look up the menu online so you can plan your order calmly. If one friend is always the catalyst for a 2am finish, then maybe they're not the right person to hang out with when you need to focus on feeling good.

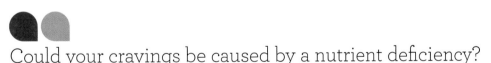

Could your cravings be caused by a nutrient deficiency?

The idea goes that you're driven to binge because your body is lacking in a vital nutrient [14]. An obsession with chocolate suggests a lack of magnesium, the muscle relaxant; salty cravings have been linked to calcium deficiencies; a non-specific desire for fatty foods may be attributed to not eating enough healthy fats; while cravings for meat may be related to low iron levels. If you binge consistently, then something is consistently wrong in your diet. So experiment—eat a little more magnesium-rich leafy greens, calcium-packed cheese, healthy fats like avocado or iron-charged steak for a week.

Mostly green: you're a secret eater

Though you may exert a lot of control around food in front of people, when no one is watching you have very different habits. Secret eating can happen when you don't eat enough in the day—your body will rebel and force you to eat in the evening. That urge can build up to the point where you're trapped in the throes of an all-out binge.

When I'm alone I can eat whatever and however I like

If I felt good about eating a giant tub of ice cream, I'd do it in front of my friends

I was really restrained earlier, so it's OK to eat all this now

Just because I turned down food earlier doesn't give me carte blanche to binge now. My body only knows what I do eat, not what I don't

Dismiss sabotaging secret eating thoughts and listen to your body

OVERCOME SECRET EATING

It doesn't matter whether no one's watching or a thousand people gawp at you eating a whole loaf of bread, because either way, you're eating way beyond your body's needs. Overeating is overeating.

Prevent slipping into secret eating by eating at regular 4-hour intervals during the day and knowing the right things that satisfy you physically and emotionally. It's vital for you to eat a balance of food groups, so as well as getting essential nutrients from protein, vegetables and healthy fats, be sure to include some carbs or even dessert. Eliminating sweet things may make you feel like you're missing out, which can lead to secret eating. Have a little—just a little—of something you really like at each meal, so it stops unhealthy urges to eat more of it later when you're alone. You've actually got more willpower when you eat your sweet treat at the table as part of your meal. Why? Because other foods will buffer the insulin rollercoaster and you'll eat more mindfully with utensils and crockery than if you slouch on the sofa and trough from a package.

Is the urge to binge rising inside you like a wave about to break? You're still in time to consciously acknowledge your behaviour in the moment before binge mentality takes over. Switch the light on to raise your awareness—darkness intensifies secret eating. As you see your food in front of you and watch your hand go to your mouth, you'll eat less. Give yourself visual clues, too: leave debris on your plate and don't bury packaging in the bin. When we have evidence of what we've consumed, we eat 28% less [15].

Now you've aced the practical, we've got to deal with the deeper emotional issue: shame. When we feel ashamed, we're driven to eat well beyond what our body needs, even though such behaviour can make us feel weaker and out of control [16]. Use the practical tips above to put the brake on secret eating before it starts. If you slip up, the recovery remedies on page 39 will help you move on from a binge.

FOOD DIARY TIP FOR SECRET EATERS

No one but you is going to see your journal, so don't hold back. Keep your food diary close by and live-blog what you eat as you eat it. The greater your acknowledgment of what's happening, the better handle you'll have on secret eating.

Draw a line

If you find it hard to stop before you see the bottom of the package, draw a line to mark your portion size. That visible marker on a giant food package is like a subconscious red light that stops you overeating [17]. Look up the portion size on the package and get busy with your magic marker.

Mostly purple: you're an accidental eater

The free bag of pretzels that came with your lunchtime meal deal, a leftover sandwich from a meeting in the boardroom, a handful of grated cheese while you're cooking dinner … oops, you ate it again. If you accidentally pick at food all day, you will lack energy, gain weight and wonder why you feel so bad.

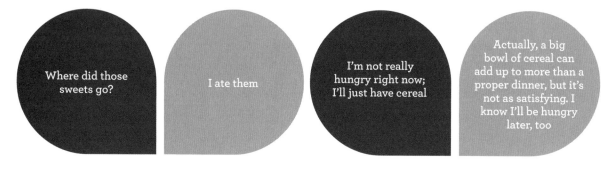

Where did those sweets go?

I ate them

I'm not really hungry right now; I'll just have cereal

Actually, a big bowl of cereal can add up to more than a proper dinner, but it's not as satisfying. I know I'll be hungry later, too

Dismiss sabotaging ideas about accidental eating and listen to your body

OVERCOME ACCIDENTAL EATING

The big problem with accidental munching is that you load up on calories without the psychological satisfaction of eating. This means you're always fighting the urge to eat more.

Here's what to do: hold up your hand and make a fist. That is the actual size of your stomach. Before you eat any food, compare it to the size of your fist, then ask yourself if it will comfortably fit in your belly.

As an accidental eater, you may find it easier to enforce a snack embargo than trying to monitor the bits of that and bites of this that pass your lips every day. Focus on meals and think in advance about what you'd like to eat. As you discovered earlier in this chapter, it's clinically proven that anticipation makes any food from carrot sticks to chocolate cake taste better and feel more emotionally satisfying, too.

As you eat, insert pause points to slow down your meal. Lay down your utensils between mouthfuls and observe the color, fragrance, texture and taste of each new forkful. The more alert your senses, the less likely you'll eat to the point you feel uncomfortable.

Outsmart the "because it's there" Everest effect. Visually sweep the room for temptation and make a mental note not to have the cookie sitting beside your teacup. Tuck it under your saucer—you're less likely to eat it if you can't see it. As for leftovers, even a forkful of pasta or a surplus fishfinger from your child's dinner can be stored in a small plastic box, so don't worry about wastage. Your body is not a dustbin.

FOOD DIARY TIP FOR ACCIDENTAL EATERS

Keep a photographic food journal. Whipping out your smartphone before chowing down helps you pause and register what you're doing [18]. Seeing your food on screen also breaks your subconscious hand-to-mouth action.

Break your emotional eating habits—for good

Now you've unpicked your emotional eating, all that's left is the shadow of a bad habit. If you believe you're capable of change, you can rewire your brain with positive habits instead [19]. As you learn new skills—like managing your stress by getting fresh air, not wolfing down a bag of sickly marshmallows—your brain cells develop new connections between them. Neuroscientists have found that when people practise new skills, the area of the brain responsible for those skills actually enlarges, and your brain speeds up its production of new nerve cells. In other words, you're no longer a slave to emotional eating. You are free.

Chocolate + self-control = you
It is humanly possible to eat just a little. Seriously

The number one craving can be a challenge to handle. We like to believe that chocolate is the cure for tiredness, headaches, heartache and every kind of stress imaginable. Though chocolate is one of the most delicious things ever, eating too much of it can make us feel bad.

You might find it easier to abstain altogether because one piece of chocolate opens the dopamine floodgates, and this hormone sends a signal to your brain that's like a siren screaming MORE! MORE! MORE! But there's also a huge body of research to back up what your grandmother told you: eating a little of what you crave does you good.

To enjoy chocolate and feel good, select the dark, organic variety. Cocoa is the ingredient that really does the business because it is rich in antioxidant flavonoids that can improve heart health [20]. Choose a 70% bar as it has more cocoa than sugar, which is ultimately more satisfying.

The best time to enjoy that chocolate is at the end of your meal so your hunger is already satisfied. You've filled your body with feelgood nutrients; you don't need to eat more. Think of that square as punctuation that seals your meal with a smile. Savour that square slowly. Feel the creaminess melt on your tongue. Taste the dark, cocoa-y loveliness and feel good about yourself. Easy? It is now.

Being hydrated will help cut cravings, big time.
Here's how to make your water more interesting

Swipe a wedge of lemon around the rim of your glass, as if you were making a cocktail. **Chop slices of strawberry** into your ice-cube tray and freeze. **Infuse your water with cucumber and mint,** as if you were in a spa. **Drink bubbles**—sparkling water still counts. **Hit boiling point**—herbal tea definitely counts. **Blend** a green juice. **Eat your water**—cucumber, radishes and celery are all 95% water. **Add alkalining chlorophyll drops,** which can help your blood cells carry oxygen around your body.

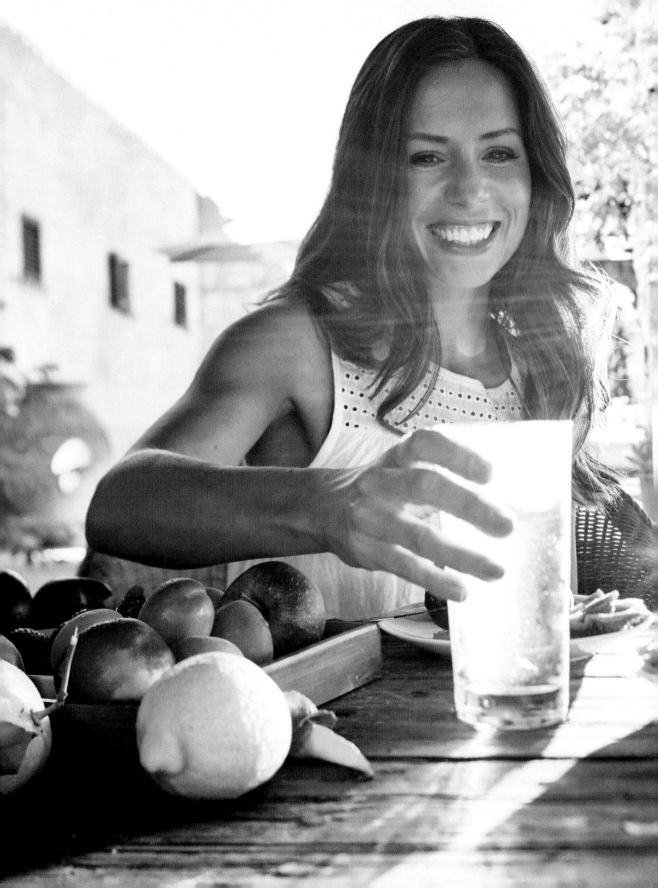

SNACKS WITH FEELGOOD SUPERPOWERS

When you've got more than 4 hours between meals, you may well need a bite to keep you feeling good. These snacks all have natural relaxing, energising and brain-boosting properties, so you'll stay calm and keep your can-do attitude all day long

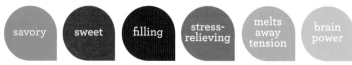

savory · sweet · filling · stress-relieving · melts away tension · brain power

1 **Air-popped popcorn** has fewer calories than a banana, twice as many antioxidants as any fruit, plus twice as much fiber as prunes [21]. Air-pop yours and add a pinch of sea salt, or sprinkle with cinnamon to satisfy your sweet tooth. Even better, top your popcorn with cayenne pepper, which contains craving-killing capsaicin.

2 **Peanut butter-filled celery canoes** are quick to prep: simply load celery sticks with nut butter. Protein and fat from the PB are satisfying, while celery is refreshing. Together, you've got a crunchy, munchy feelgood hit.

3 **Cashews and blueberries** are a winning combination of protein, fat and the brain-boosting antioxidant anthocyanin. This sweet-and-savory snack balances blood sugar and is particularly relaxing: the nuts deliver anxiety-easing zinc [22], while the purple pearls are high in vitamin C, which is an important weapon against stress. Choose raw, unsalted cashews.

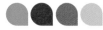

Full-fat Greek yogurt contains potassium, a natural muscle relaxant. Potassium is also used to create digestive enzymes, which break down food so it passes through your gut without causing trouble. This creamy treat has twice the protein of regular yogurt, so it keeps you feeling pleasantly full for longer.

Almond milk is naturally sweet, deliciously nutty and high in tryptophan. This calming amino acid is what your brain then turns into serotonin—the neurotransmitter responsible for regulating your appetite and mood. Add a scoop of protein powder for the perfect post-workout snack.

Dark chocolate is sweet without de-stabilising your blood sugar or messing with your metabolism. The 70% cocoa squares can improve blood flow and regulate your stress hormone, too.

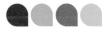

Coconut milk yogurt is delicious and also a dairy-free source of fiber, which means less risk of bloating. This healthy energy hit will keep you craving-free for hours.

Crudités and hummus are such a great go-to for protein plus veggie goodness and fiber. This snack is surprisingly portable—try putting a spoonful of hummus in a glass jar and standing sticks of carrot, red pepper and sugar snap peas in it.

Apple slices with walnut butter, yummy. Fat makes humble apple more satisfying and walnuts are a decent source of omega-3s, which are great for helping your brain handle stress.

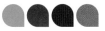

Hard-boiled eggs keep for a week in the fridge. Nature's protein ball is also a good source of choline, which improves brain function.

GIVE THESE SNACKS THE SLIP

You know obvious culprits like cookies cause your body to crash, but these five healthy-seeming snacks are all mostly sugar, too

❶ Trail mix ❷ Flavored, fat-free yogurt ❸ Granola bar ❹ Protein bars ❺ Dried fruits like dates, cranberries and mango

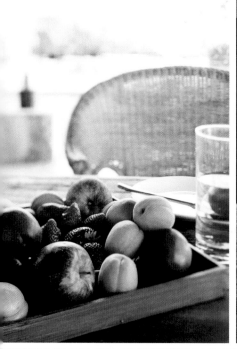
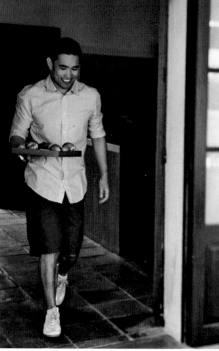
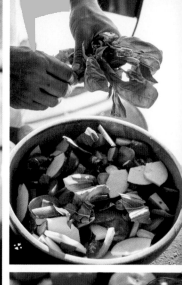
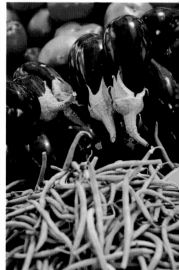

SHOP YOURSELF HAPPY

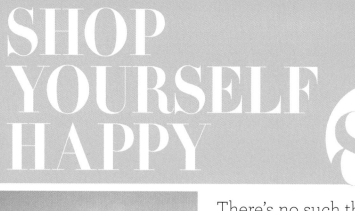

There's no such thing as no-strings shopping. What you put in your cart has a direct link to what you put in your body

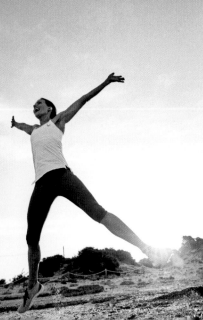
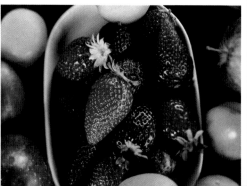
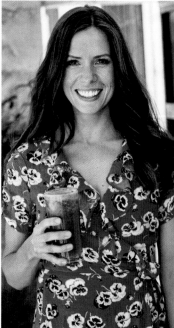

SMART SUPERMARKET STRATEGIES
Save stress, time and your sanity with these five moves

1 Make a menu. A mere list won't cut it—after all, how many times have you set out with one and gone home with a bag of extras? Plan a full menu for the week, then you'll only pick the necessary ingredients for making those meals, which is good news for your bank balance, too. If you're prone to throwing an additional this or that into your cart regardless, buy online. It's easier to resist purchasing junk food when you know you can't eat it straight away.

2 Schedule to shop after dinner. Rushing around the supermarket when you're desperate for dinner on your way home from work means you're easy prey for refined carbs that promise instant energy. Get your groceries when you are fed and watered because then you'll have the willpower to make healthy choices. Schedule 30 minutes to shop when you're not rushed, so you have time to evaluate your healthiest options.

3 Use a cart, not a basket. In theory, a basket gives you less wiggle room for making dodgy decisions. In reality, carrying a basket means you're more likely to make unhealthy purchases. The arm-flexor contraction made shoppers choose products that provide instant gratification—unconsciously picking up sugary products to compensate for the physical discomfort [1].

4 Load your cart as you would your plate. That means 80% of everything you buy is vegetables, fruit, fish, lean meat, complex carbohydrates and healthy fats. Use the main section of the cart for all your healthy produce, then flip out the child seat and place your 20% of cheesecake, curly fries or preferred treats there.

5 Shop once or twice a week. One big shop for staples plus a top-up cart dash for fresh fruit and vegetables means your feelgood intentions won't be ruined by an empty cupboard or a bag of soggy salad. Try to do your biggest shopping at the weekend when you have more time to cook, then another after dinner on Wednesday evening, when supermarkets are typically quietest. It gives you the best chance of going in and getting what you need without feeling like only a tub of double-fudge ice cream will stop you committing murder in the bagging area.

Planning your feelgood menu
This menu will satisfy your appetite and your wallet, as it makes over your leftovers into even more yummy meals

SUNDAY

- **Protein pancakes with berries—** blend 1 cup cottage cheese, ½ cup oats or rye flakes, 2 eggs and a shake of cinnamon, then fry for 2 minutes each side in a medium hot pan
- **Roast chicken** with roast sweet potatoes, carrot and beetroot, plus purple-sprouting broccoli and Chinese cabbage
- **Slow-cooked lamb tagine** with quinoa, butternut squash and a zesty green salad

NOTES Cook on a big scale! You can make over your leftovers with chicken salad on Monday, Tuesday night's Thai curry, chicken soup (with the stock) for lunch on Wednesday, then roast carrots and sweet potato wedges with your steak for a quick midweek dinner. While your chicken is in the oven, halve a butternut squash, rub it with butter and salt, and bake that, too— then you're set for your evening meal and Monday's dinner as well. At dinner, throw extra lamb into your tagine for Tuesday's lamb mezze lunch. Your quinoa will come in handy for Friday's sushi, too.

MONDAY

- **Greek yogurt** with blueberries, raspberries and strawberries
- **Chicken salad** with tomatoes, cucumber, watercress, radishes and chunks of roast beetroot
- **Roast butternut squash soup** with fresh chilies

NOTES For extra flavor, stir stock from yesterday's roast chicken into your butternut squash soup.

TUESDAY

- **Boiled eggs** and rye bread sticks
- **Lamb mezze** with hummus, sugar snap peas, radishes, avocado and tomatoes
- **Thai chicken curry** with onions, garlic, ginger, red peppers, sugar snap peas and kale, served on a bed of coriander-infused cauli rice

NOTES How to make cauliflower rice? Easy. Pulse the florets in your blender until they reach a rice-like consistency, then heat on the stove with a tablespoon of coconut oil and freshly torn coriander. Sauté until the cauliflower dries out and begins to go golden brown.

WEDNESDAY

- **Blended berry bowl** with berries, banana, avocado, pumpkin seeds
- **Chicken soup**
- **Steak and sweet potato wedges** with roast carrots, purple-sprouting broccoli, green beans and mushrooms

NOTES Thanks to the fact you've already roasted your carrots and sweet potato wedges, you can warm them through so they're ready in the time it takes your steak to sizzle. Cook a large steak, rubbing on a little chili powder and pinch of cayenne on half of it for your taco lunch tomorrow.

THURSDAY

- **Banana oatmeal** with almonds
- **Steak tacos**—use lettuce as taco shells and pile them with steak, kidney beans, your favorite veggies, a little leftover cauli rice and a sprinkle of cheese
- **Rainbow frittata** with cheddar, kale, asparagus, Chinese cabbage and any other veggies you like—the more the merrier

NOTES Steak tacos are a surprisingly portable lunch hit. Wrap your steak strips in foil, then box up your vegetables and assemble your tacos at your desk.

FRIDAY

- **Rye toast** with cashew nut butter
- **Prawn sushi futomaki**, basically a big nori wrap rolled with avocado, cucumber, radishes and sugar snap peas. Use quinoa instead of white rice
- **Tuna steaks** and multi-hued roast veg. And banana ice cream, because it's practically the weekend

NOTES Actually, banana ice cream is a great everyday treat. Just peel a banana, break it into chunks and freeze it. A quick blend and you've got a rich, creamy ice cream. Flavor yours with nut butter or drizzle it with melted dark chocolate and you'll never look back.

SATURDAY

- **Smoked salmon** with asparagus, tomatoes, avocado and arugula on rye
- **Salad Niçoise** with soft-boiled eggs, last night's tuna, olives, green beans and a medley of salad leaves
- **Vegetable chili** with your five-a-day in one dish. This is a great meal for using up leftover veg. Creamy avocado guacamole and coriander on top is a must

NOTES You've eaten well all week, which leaves room for life's little indulgences.

 Take 15 minutes to plan your menu for the week and set up a healthy shopping list online

DRINKS

- **Home-blended green juice**—Ginger, lemon, cucumber, spinach, celery and a dollop of nut butter is our feelgood go-to. Add an apple, berries or half a banana if you prefer yours sweeter
- **Sparkling water,** for when good old tap water activates your "bored" alarm
- **Camomile, mint, ginger or any herbal tea**
- **Coffee and English breakfast tea**

SNACKS

- **Dark chocolate**
- **Apple slices dipped in nut butter**
- **Berries and almonds**
- **Hard-boiled eggs**
- **Crudités and hummus**
- **Cheese on cucumber rounds**
- **Olives**
- **Celery canoes with nut butter**

Shopping list

Fresh produce:
* Apples
* Asparagus
* Avocados
* Bananas
* Beetroot
* Blueberries
* Butternut squash
* Carrots
* Cauliflower
* Celery
* Chillies
* Chinese cabbage
* Coriander
* Cucumber
* Garlic
* Ginger
* Green beans
* Kale
* Lemons
* Little gem lettuce
* Mushrooms
* Olives
* Onions
* Purple sprouting broccoli
* Radishes
* Raspberries
* Red peppers
* Salad bags of arugula, watercress and spinach
* Strawberries
* Sugar snap peas
* Sweet potatoes
* Tomatoes

For your fridge:
* Butter
* Cashew nut butter
* Cottage cheese
* Cheddar
* Chicken (whole)
* Eggs
* Greek yogurt
* Hummus
* Lamb neck fillets
* Milk
* Prawns (cooked)
* Smoked salmon
* Sparkling water
* Steak
* Tuna steak

For your cupboards:
* Almonds
* Chocolate (choose a bar with 70% cocoa)
* Chopped tomatoes
* Coconut oil (for stir-frying)
* Coffee
* Kidney beans
* Nori sheets
* Oats/rye flakes
* Olive oil (for dressing salads)
* Pumpkin seeds
* Quinoa
* Rye bread
* Teas, like green, mint, camomile or English breakfast

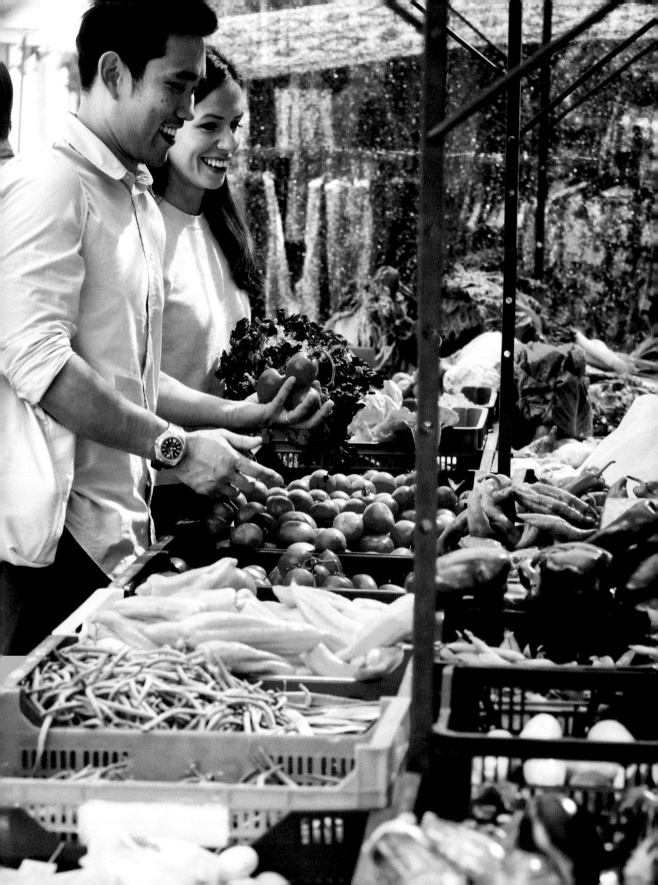

Prioritize your staples. Though many foods only contain low levels of pesticides, they add up when you eat them every day.

Look out for organic goods close to their sell-by date on the "reduced" shelf

If your meat isn't organic, trim off the fat because that's where most of the toxins are stored. If your meat is organic, eat the whole thing

Do you really need to eat organic?
Your guide to when it's worth splashing out and where you can save [2]

FRUIT AND VEGETABLES

Buy organic: pre-prepared salad leaves, grapes, nectarines and peaches
Maybe: apples, apricots, broad beans, cabbage, kiwi fruit, leeks, lettuce, onions, peppers, rhubarb and tomatoes
Save your money: avocados, pineapple, asparagus, peas, eggplant, broccoli and sweet potatoes

GRAINS

Buy organic: oats
Maybe: wheat products like bread
Save your money: corn on the cob, spelt, rye, brown rice

ANIMAL PRODUCTS

Buy organic: chicken, eggs, bacon, ham, sausages and other processed pork products
Maybe: cheese, butter and ice cream
Save your money: milk and yogurt

WHY DIET FOOD MAKES YOU FAT

People who understand food labels weigh 9lb less than those who don't [3]. Here's what you need to know

"Low fat" often means "high sugar". When fat is extracted, manufacturers have to replace it with sugar or artificial sweeteners, because otherwise processed food tastes like pulped cardboard. Without the fat, your body doesn't release leptin, the hormone that tells your brain you're full.
Result: you keep eating. Sugar is far more fattening than fat itself.

Look at the order of ingredients because manufacturers are legally bound to put the largest one first. If, as on a protein bar, the first, second and third ingredients are different varieties of sugars (sucrose, fructose and saccharin), then you know it's more of a "sugar bar" than a "protein bar".

"Diet" drinks actually make us crave more sugar [4]—Instead of being a risk-free sweet fix, artifically sweetened fizzy drinks are believed to increase your risk of becoming obese, having high blood sugar and developing metabolic syndrome, which is a key precursor of heart disease and diabetes. Switch to sparkling water if you love the fizz, infuse it with fresh fruit if you want more flavor, and load it with ice for a wake-up.

Don't worry if you genuinely love the odd "diet" soda. They're not complete no-nos, they're just not everyday items if you want to feel good. Should the odd can of diet soda appear in your hands, just try to be more mindful of what you eat on those days.

Don't feel bad because you didn't have the right information. Now you know, you can make better decisions for your body

Think outside the supermarket
Ditch your cart to find feelgood food at a fraction of the price

BUTCHER

- As the 2013 horsemeat scandal proves, trust is essential when it comes to meat. Here, you can trace exactly where your meat came from. Your butcher can tell you exactly what's in your sausages because he made them himself.

- Cheaper cuts of meat such as beef brisket and lamb shoulder are delicious when cooked in a long, slow heat.

- Squeamish? The butcher can prepare offal so it's ready to cook. Oxtail is an excellent source of flu-fighting zinc, liver is best when you're low on energy as it's high in iron, and heart is an exceptionally lean form of protein. Oh, and it's all phenomenal value.

- Most butchers give away bones so you can make your own delicious stock for soups, casseroles and curries.

- Go regularly and you'll build a relationship with your butcher, which means discounts.

FISHMONGER

- Your local fishmonger only sells fresh, local, seasonal fish, and can tell you how to get the best from them. For example, lobster and crab taste best in summer, and you'll get the best price on mussels and oysters in early spring.

- This is the place to buy more sustainable species like black cod, chub and spiny dogfish, which are particularly high in omega-3.

- But if you still want salmon, you can save money buying a whole side of it here. Chop it into portions for your freezer.

- Most fishmongers will prepare the fish for you at no extra cost.

VEGETABLE BOX DELIVERY

- Great for veg you've never heard of like black salsify and romanesque cauliflower—and recipes for them.

- Can supply locally grown salad, even in winter.

- The big players in the vegetable box business also deliver meat, milk, eggs, bread, muesli, baby food and wine. All the essentials!

FARMERS' MARKET/FARM SHOP

- You can buy food that's virtually organic without the price tag. It takes 7 years for land to be classified organic, but chat to the farmer and you may find his produce is grown in a healthy, sustainable and environmentally friendly way.

- Locally-grown produce is harvested at peak ripeness, so you eat it when nutrients are at their very best.

- Some fruits and vegetables in supermarkets are up to 12 weeks old. Farm produce doesn't sit around in a storeroom, so it stays fresh for longer, which means less wastage.

- There's no middleman, so the savings get passed on to you.

ETHNIC MINIMARKET

- A great place to pick up inexpensive herbs and spices in bulk.

- Boost your immune system by experimenting with unusual vegetables. Try oca, a South American yam that's an excellent source of potassium and iron, or the German root vegetable kohlrabi, which contains more vitamin C than oranges.

- Source global health foods, like the Korean pickle kimchi, which contains a powerful probiotic that's great for your gut [5].

HEALTH FOOD SHOP

- If you want to be extra careful about hidden sugars, the selection of muesli, protein powder and probiotic yogurts is health heaven.

- Vegetarian or vegan? Here's where to find a huge range of tofu and other plant protein, like tempeh. Like tofu it's made from soybeans, but it's less processed so contains more fiber and protein. You can even buy vegan protein powder made from pea or hemp.

- The artisan bread range is enormous: choose from buckwheat, rye, spelt, yeast-free and every gluten-free variety imaginable.

- Good health food shops sell pasta made from corn, spelt or even spinach and beetroot instead of wheat.

- Stock up on alternatives to the humble peanut butter, such as cashew, macadamia or almond nut butter.

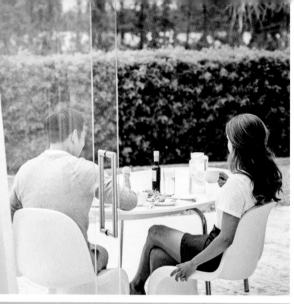

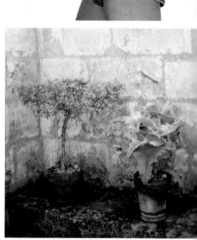

HOW TO BE HEALTHY IN THE REAL WORLD 9

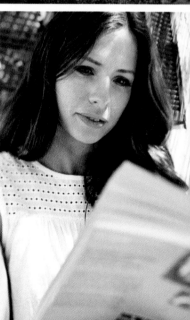

What feels easy at home can be challenging when you're out and about, rarely more than 10 feet from temptation. Use these feelgood grids to stay focused

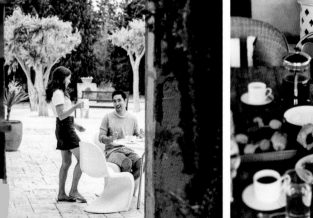

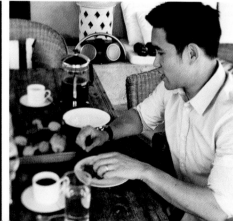

We take cues about what and how much to eat from our surroundings, which explains why you often find yourself putting food into your mouth that makes you feel bad

Trying to find any vaguely healthy food in, say, a cocktail party or a movie, means the odds are stacked against you—eating on the run usually means overdoing fast food, unhealthy fats and not consuming enough protein, complex carbohydrates and vegetables [1].

Don't panic: this chapter will swing the odds forever in your favor. There is always a feelgood option. And it's never a dusty rice cake with sloppy cottage cheese; it's tasty, satisfying food that makes you feel really good.

Some situations are best avoided. You're very unlikely to find a nourishing, satisfying meal in a fast-food joint, so don't stress looking for one. Go elsewhere.

You may worry you're being judged when you say "no thanks" to cookies or as you ask for no croutons and dressing on the side. And you probably are: we admire people with willpower. What's the worst someone will think—that you're a healthy person who knows what makes you feel good? You're cool with that.

Sometimes friends and family may try to push food on you that will make you feel bloated, uncomfortable or regretful. They don't realize they're making your life difficult; feeding is just the way some people are conditioned to show love. Accept their niceness and concern, make them feel appreciated, but do what makes you feel good. It helps to have a line ready to go: "This looks delicious, thank you, but I had a big lunch. You enjoy it."

Some people may be jealous of how easy it is for you to eat good food while they battle their own demons. That's their issue. Focus on what's right for you.

Things calm down when friends and family accept this is your new normal. What's more, healthy eaters (that's you!) subconsciously influence weight loss among people close to them [2]. So when others notice the change in you—your energy, your bounce, your body—they may want to know your secret to feeling good.

 Eating out? Take 15 minutes to review the menu so you can pick your feelgood option

THE FEELGOOD GUIDE TO
EATING OUT

Restaurants make money by tricking you into eating more than you want to. Here's your seven-step good-time guarantee

1 Download the menu so you can choose what to order in advance
The more you anticipate a meal, the more it tickles your tastebuds.

2 Never go out ravenous
We've all demolished the bread basket and regretted it, right? So power up with complex carbs like granola, hummus or carrot crudités before going out so you're pleasantly hungry as you order, not starving.

3 Choose a softly-lit spot
Bright colors stimulate your appetite as well as your eyes and can increase the amount you eat by 25% [3]. Ask to be seated in a candlelit corner where you can relax.

4 Wear an extra layer
Why do restaurants crank up the air-con? Because a 5°C reduction in temperature increases food consumption by nearly 20% [4]. Leptin, a hormone that controls your appetite, is slower to kick in when your body temperature is low.

5 Forgo the freebies
If you're having carbs with your meal, say no thanks to the bread basket now—too much of a good thing can make you feel rotten. A handful of olives are a better bet than bread. Choose black over green as dark olives contain 50% less sodium.

6 Order first
You won't get swayed by your friend who goes for the creamy pasta—you'll order the food that makes you feel good.

7 Delay drinking
Alcohol on an empty stomach encourages you to eat more [5]. Booze makes everything a bit fuzzy, including your body's "I'm full" signals. Give yourself a fighting chance by sipping sparkling water until your food arrives (it makes you feel fuller than plain old tap water), then enjoy a glass of wine with dinner.

If you're hungry:

starter + main

If you want to lose weight:

starter + another starter as your main

If you have a sweet tooth:

main + share a dessert

If you want to lose weight and you have a sweet tooth:

starter as a main + share a dessert

Be a feelgood dinner party guest

Going to a friend's house for dinner is 80% about the company, and only 20% about the food. So focus on being with your friends and relax; there's no need to stress about what you're going to eat.

As your host dishes up, say yes to lots of vegetables, praise the cooking and if you don't like the inevitable mound of white rice or potatoes, just leave it to the side of your plate. Chew your food mindfully and use the fact that you're engaged in conversation to put down your knife and fork between mouthfuls—this allows time for your fullness gauge to register.

You could offer to bring fresh berries for dessert, but it's totally fine to enjoy some pudding, especially if it's home-made. A few mouthfuls of even the most decadent pie in the world won't blow your plan. If you're enjoying the food, take time to relish every mouthful and feel the flavors melt on your tongue. When you've had enough, lay down your spoon and say yes please to some peppermint or camomile tea.

EAT OUT THE FEELGOOD WAY

FEELS BAD	FEELS OK	FEELS GOOD
Steak and fries		
Grain-fed American steak with blue cheese sauce and fries	Grass-fed free-range steak with mushroom sauce and oven-baked wedges	Organic grass-fed steak in its natural state with broccoli, peas and sweet potato wedges
Chicken		
Chicken Milanese or any other breaded, fried chicken dish with fries	Corn-fed chicken with mashed potato and glazed vegetables	Organic roast chicken with green beans, purple sprouting broccoli and kale
Lamb		
Shepherd's pie	Lamb tagine with couscous	Braised lamb shank with peas, mangetout and cabbage
Pork		
Sausages and mashed potatoes with gravy, or pulled pork	Ham, egg and oven-baked fries	Grilled tenderloin pork chops with green vegetables
Fish		
Battered fish and chips	Deepwater fish like tuna and swordfish. Though they are nutritious, these species often contain mercury so don't eat them more than once a week	Steamed, grilled or barbecued salmon or mackerel. Oily fish is the most nutritious, especially served with vegetables
Seafood		
Deep-fried calamari or crab cakes with a side of fries	Prawns or any factory-farmed seafood served in a creamy sauce with a side of oven-baked fries	Lobster, oysters, scallops, mussels or razor clams served in nothing but butter and lemon, with spinach, green beans or broccoli on the side
Pizza		
Stuffed-crust pizza pie with pepperoni and extra cheese	Italian-style thin-crust pizza with chicken, mozzarella and peppers	Half a thin-crust pizza and half a green salad, shared with a friend. The Fiorentina with egg, cheese, black olives and spinach is perfect

FEELS BAD	FEELS OK	FEELS GOOD
Pasta		
Carbonara, or any pasta in a creamy sauce	Bolognese, or any pasta with some meat or fish protein in a tomato-based sauce	A starter portion of your favorite pasta, or just the sauce with salad
Chinese		
Sweet-and-sour pork with special-fried rice	Peking rotisserie duck with egg-fried rice	Stir-fried beef in black bean sauce with broccoli
Japanese		
Chicken katsu curry with white rice, or any tempura dish	Chicken or salmon teriyaki with brown rice	Salmon or mackerel sashimi with seaweed and miso soup
Indian		
Korma, masala, pasanda or any creamy curry with rice, naan bread, poppadoms and mango chutney	Rogan josh, jalfrezi, bhuna or any curry in a tomato-based sauce, with only one high-carb side dish like naan or rice (not both!)	Chicken or fish tandoori with spinach sag aloo, okra and dahl on the side
Thai		
Deep-fried prawns with coconut rice and prawn crackers	Red or green curry with steamed rice	Grilled chicken satay or prawn stir-fry with spicy spinach
Mexican		
Pork taco with refried beans, cheese, sour cream and cheesy-topped nachos	Beef burrito in a whole wheat wrap with cheese and salad	Chicken in a lettuce-wrap burrito with pinto beans and freshly made guacamole
Beef burger		
Fast-food burgers contain as little as 2% meat [6] and are served in tasteless, processed buns. Add-ons to avoid: fries, deep-fried onions, processed cheese slices, mayonnaise, coleslaw, bacon and ketchup	Ground beef in a freshly made bun, with mustard and thick-cut fries, plus a side salad	Pure organic steak burger on a freshly baked open bun, topped with avocado and kimchi pickles, plus sweet potato wedges and a green side salad

FEELS BAD	FEELS OK	FEELS GOOD
Chicken burger		
Deep-fried chicken burger made from reformed meat in batter or breadcrumbs	Grilled chicken burger, which is recognisably meat	Organic grilled chicken burger that's definitely real meat
Veggie burger		
Deep-fried veggie burger that's mostly potato or synthetic meat substitute	Grilled veggie burger	Portobello mushroom burger in a stack of grilled peppers, and eggplant: a pure veggie burger
Fries		
Shoestring fries with ketchup and mayonnaise	Pan-fried potato wedges with table salt and vinegar	Oven-baked sweet potato wedges with sea salt
Sunday roast		
Pork with crackling, instant gravy, roast white potatoes, and honey-glazed vegetables	Free-range chicken, beef or lamb with freshly made gravy, new potatoes and two kinds of vegetables	Organic chicken, beef or lamb in its natural state with sweet potatoes and a medley of green vegetables like broccoli, peas, kale, green beans, mange tout and Brussels sprouts

Just because you can cram an entire canapé into your mouth doesn't mean you should— be mindful.

THE FEELGOOD GUIDE TO
CANAPÉS

Yes, canapés can make a healthy dinner.
Here's the smartest selection

FEELS BAD	FEELS OK	FEELS GOOD
Meat Hot dogs, chicken tenders, spring rolls or mini pasties	Mini burgers or marinated chicken drumsticks	Chicken skewers, lamb kofta or open-faced mini burgers
Fish Fish sticks, filo-wrapped prawns, deep-fried fish cakes, or mini fish and chips	Smoked salmon blinis or sushi with white rice	Sashimi, sushi with brown rice, king prawns or smoked salmon minus the blinis
Vegetarian Deep-fried spring rolls or samosas	Oven-baked spring rolls or samosas, or open-faced filo "parcels" with feta cheese	Vietnamese spring rolls or samosas, if they are made with rice paper, not pastry
Cheese Breaded, deep-fried brie or cheese straws	Baked brie, cheddar, manchego or blue cheese	Goat's cheese or mozzarella skewers are your healthiest options
Dippers Chips scooping creamy dip like Thousand Island dressing, or a sugary dip like sweet chili jam	Pita chips dunked in hummus	Raw crudités dipped in fresh guacamole or salsa
Nuts Roasted, salted peanuts	Raw cashews, or any other variety of unadulterated nut	Raw pistachios—shelling them means you eat more mindfully

Alcohol ain't that healthy, however you pour it. But you probably want a drink anyway. So what's the best way to handle it?

Alcohol increases levels of your stress hormone, cortisol, which encourages your body to store fat. Before you uncork the bottle, book a calming yoga class for tomorrow. It's one of the healthiest ways to cut cravings for unhealthy stress-relievers.

Leave your glass on the table as you pour, and you'll serve yourself 12% less without feeling short-changed [7].

Drink from a heavy glass. We associate them with better quality, so we drink more slowly in order to appreciate our beverages [8].

Having a glass of red wine with dinner is practically medicinal. Its enzymes are proven to balance blood sugar and drinking it with red meat reduces cancer-causing carcinogens [9].

When blending your own cocktails, use alcohol with a lower proof to save calories and have a clearer head tomorrow morning. Fresh fruit, sparkling water, lemon and green juice make the healthiest mixers.

Avoid mixing alcohol with energy drinks. Combining depressants (booze) with stimulants (caffeine) makes you feel simultaneously wired and tired, and the result is messy. In fact, mixing alcohol with energy drinks increases the risks associated with alcohol and is worse for you than drinking alone [10].

Mixing drinks combines different types of congeners, which is a fancy way of saying your body has to work harder to fight those toxins. Stick to one order.

Want to feel giddy on less booze? Drink bubbles. Fizzy mixers make you tipsy faster, as the gas helps push alcohol through your gut into your bloodstream [11].

Prefer to pace yourself? Listen to soft music with a slow beat. Fast, loud music dulls the taste senses, which means you'll drink more [12].

Try going to sleep on your left side as this position is the most restorative. One night of boozing reduces deep REM sleep and cuts 30 minutes off your total sleep, which drains your energy. A pillow propped behind you should keep you from rolling over.

What does "moderate consumption" really mean?

According to the Dietary Guidelines for Americans, moderate alcohol consumption is defined as having up to one drink per day for a woman, and up to two for men.

But, y'know, on the rare occasions you forget what moderate means, just remember your feelgood pick-me-ups: gentle exercise, extra vegetables, plenty of water, home cooking, complex carbs over refined ones and early nights.

FEELS BAD	FEELS OK	FEELS GOOD
Champagne		
Kir Royal—the crème de cassis is extra sugar you're unlikely to burn off	Buck's Fizz with fresh orange juice—though you're halving the alcohol, be aware you are replacing it with sugar	"Ultra Brut" translates as "no added sugar" in the champagne world, which means less calories in any language. Champagne cuts through fatty foods, so helping digestion. What's more, typically small champagne flutes mean you're unlikely to drink too much unawares
Red wine		
Mulled wine is just red wine with extra sugar. The additional mulling spices can't redeem that	Regular red wine contains the antioxidant resveratrol, which is linked to a lower risk of heart disease [13]	Organic red wine is made without herbicides, pesticides and fungicides, which means a less toxic hangover. Drink yours Argentinian-style (topped up with water) to prevent a sore head
White or rosé wine		
White or pink lemonade spritzer. Sugar overload!	Normal white wine doesn't contain as much resveratrol as red because the skins are removed during processing, but it still delivers some nutrients and antioxidants	Organic white or rosé spritzer. Adding a hearty splash of soda water and ice to your glass of wine helps you stay hydrated, which means a morning-after headache is less hellish
Beer		
A pint of beer is a massive cocktail of sugar, gluten and yeast. A beer belly isn't so-called for nothing	Bottled beer, because it's portion controlled	Micro-brewed beer has less toxic additives and preservatives
Cider		
Mulled cider involves more sugar (in the form of honey and brandy) being added to an already sugary drink	A pint of cider is very high in sugar. This drink only scores a spot in the "OK" column because it doesn't have extra honey and brandy in it like mulled cider. Really, it's best avoided	Bottle of micro-brewed cider poured over a pint of ice cubes—diluting your drink will make you feel better tomorrow

FEELS BAD	FEELS OK	FEELS GOOD
Mixed spirits		
Ready-mixed drinks are the worst because they're processed, which means they're exceptionally high in sugar, preservatives and additives. Fun tonight, achy head and sore tummy tomorrow	Dark spirits like rum and whisky are high in congeners, the chemical by-products of alcohol fermentation that make a simple hangover impossible to handle. In one highbrow drunk tank study, 33% of testers who drank bourbon got a severe hangover, compared to just 3% who drank the same amount of vodka [14]. If you love dark spirits, drink them over plenty of ice	Clear spirits with water-based mixers, such as vodka with soda water and fresh lime juice, or tequila with spring water, fresh lemon and agave syrup. This is probably as clean as booze gets, especially when the alcohol is organic
Cocktails		
Creamy cocktails, like White Russians and Mudslides, and syrupy liqueur blends, like Long Island Iced Tea and Mai Tai	Clear cocktails with only one spirit mixer, such as a Margarita, Mojito or Caipirinha	Clear spirits with a single fresh herb or juice mixer, and no added sugar. Order a Mint Julep or Gin Rickey
Fruity punch		
Pimm's. The sugary lemonade is actually more damaging than the alcoholic fruit cup. Sweeten your drink with fresh strawberries and just a tiny splash of lemonade instead	Sangria—at least the red wine brings some antioxidants to the party	Sangria with orange slices, not orange juice. And when you eat the fruit, the fiber helps slow the absorption of alcohol into your bloodstream—every little helps
Digestifs		
Creamy liqueurs like eggnog and Irish cream could be the sugary tipping point at which your stomach rejects its contents	Port, brandy and cognac, served on the rocks. But beware: though they're still categorized as digestifs, they all have an adverse effect on digestion	Jägermeister. Seriously. When sipped straight, not necked in "bomb" format, this digestif isn't so bad. It boasts herbs like caraway and fennel, which genuinely do aid digestion

Memo for the morning after

Fumbling your way back up your mood curve is hard when you feel sick, tired, headachey and your willpower is at an all-time low. It helps to understand what's going on with your body, so you don't eat the entire fridge as you search for the right nutrients. Here's what's happening:

"Why do I feel so bad?"
Your brain is dehydrated. Sip some water.

"I feel sick. I need chips. And bacon. With fries'
You're craving salty food because salt forces your body to drink more water. Drinking throws your natural electrolyte balance out of whack. The more hydrated you are, the more manageable your cravings will be. Put a pinch of sea salt into your water to help your body hold on to more H20. You could also try coconut water, which naturally contains magnesium, salt and electrolytes.

"Perhaps I'll have a painkiller...'
Stop right there! Ibuprofen and paracetamol are extra toxic loads that your liver has to process, so popping a pill means alcohol stays in your system even longer.

"I have the worst taste in my mouth'
That so-bad-it's-gross taste is down to dehydration. Add a squeeze of fresh lemon or lime to cut through your bad breath and help alkalize your body after last night's booze.

"Time for breakfast. What will help?'
We often overeat with a hangover—and that's on top of the excess calories from a night's drinking. Stay balanced with detoxifying, alcohol-soaking food that gives your body the necessary protein and complex carbs to repair the damage from last night's toxic insulin overload. Try avocado and smoked salmon on rye toast, an asparagus omelette or hearty oatmeal with fresh berries and nuts.

"Coffee. Get me coffee'
Stick to one for now, as caffeine dehydrates you—it's just another thing your liver has to process. Right now, your liver is kinda busy.

"How will I make it through the day?'
Take it easy. Keep sipping water. Get plenty of fresh air to increase the oxygen in your system. Have a gentle walk. Use the 60-second headache solution on page 174 to smooth the hard edges of your hangover, then you'll be set up for a long, sound sleep. Recovery: done.

Why water helps

Alcohol suppresses an antidiuretic hormone called vasopressin that tells our kidneys to reabsorb and conserve water. The more alcohol you drink, the more the vasopressin falls, and thus the more water you lose. So that explains why you have a dry tongue and a heavy head the next day.

Consider this

If you didn't know why you felt so rough the morning after, you'd be calling an ambulance. Going over your limit can feel like a near-death experience, so be gentle on yourself.

Take 1% of your day

A leisurely 15-minute walk will speed up circulation, which means your liver will work faster to process the booze in your body.

CAN'T THINK STRAIGHT? JUST DO THIS

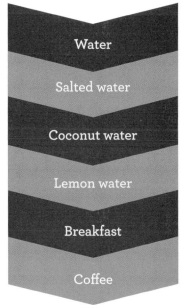

Water

Salted water

Coconut water

Lemon water

Breakfast

Coffee

THE FEELGOOD GUIDE TO
BARBECUES

The average person eats an astonishing 3,000 calories at a BBQ [15]. Whether you're manning the grill or sitting back in the sun, this cheat sheet will help you enjoy your day

FEELS BAD	FEELS OK	FEELS GOOD
Sausages		
Frankfurters are the ultimate in processed meat, made by mixing pork trimmings and the pink slurry beaten off carcasses. Revolting	Free-range sausages from your local butcher, which are typically 80% meat	Organic sausages with no rusk or filler—as good as it gets
Burgers		
Processed, intensively farmed burger that's only 60% meat—which means 40% filler	Hand-made free-range burger from your local butcher	Organic steak—heaven
Chicken		
Glazed chicken drumsticks—the skin is fatty enough to add flavor, they don't need sugar on top	Chicken thigh—remove the skin if you want to lose weight	Chicken breast is all white meat, which is the leanest cut of the bird
Fish		
Fish glazed with BBQ sauce. Why spoil fish by dousing it in sugar?	Prawn skewers, marinated in lemon juice. These are a tasty source of lean protein	Flame-grilled mackerel stuffed with lime and mango, for satisfying essential fats that boost brain function
Potatoes		
Potato salad, which is all mayonnaise and sugary white carbs	Baked potato—if you love white potatoes, eat a small one baked, with butter and salt	Sweet potato is lower GI and an excellent source of vitamin A, which boosts your immune system

FEELS BAD	FEELS OK	FEELS GOOD
Salads		
Rice salad—it sounds healthy enough, but white rice is higher on the GI scale than fries—it's sugar in another guise	Couscous salad—this is medium GI and is a good source of lean protein	Fresh rainbow salad—load with as many vegetables as you can think of and dress with lemon juice and olive oil. Always a winner
Vegetables		
No vegetables at all	Teriyaki vegetable skewers— adding soy sauce and spices is great, but sugar too? No thanks	Chargrilled pepper, mushroom and courgette skewers, dressed with olive oil
Coleslaw		
Creamy shop-bought coleslaw—sodium and mayo overload	Home-made coleslaw—at least you can control how much mayo you put in	Raw slaw, blended with either vinaigrette or a spoonful of Greek yogurt
Burger buns		
Processed white buns. Apart from having no nutritional value, these are almost as high GI as a croissant	Whole wheat buns have less sugar and more fiber than their white counterparts, which makes them more satisfying	Eating your meat in an open-faced whole wheat bun means halving the carbs
Cheese		
Processed cheese slice on a burger. Just: no	Real grated cheese on your burger. Don't melt it and it will taste even more satisfying	Mashed avocado. A layer of this healthy fat on top of your burger helps you absorb vitamins in the meat
Condiments		
Ketchup: a manufacturer's name for "red sugar"	Mustard brings out flavor in meat without sugar-bombing your body	Sauerkraut neutralizes the acid in meat and an enzyme-rich spoonful aids the digestion too
Dippers		
Chips and creamy garlic-and-herb dip—full of monosodium glutamate (MSG), which messes with your appetite-control hormone leptin. Result? You can't stop eating	Pita chips and hummus are moreish because they're a tasty combo, not because the snack spins your body out of control. Hummus is a healthy blend of plant-based fat and protein	Crudités like carrots, cucumber, peppers and sugar snap peas, dipped in fresh spicy guacamole. Brings a whole new meaning to "skinny dipping"

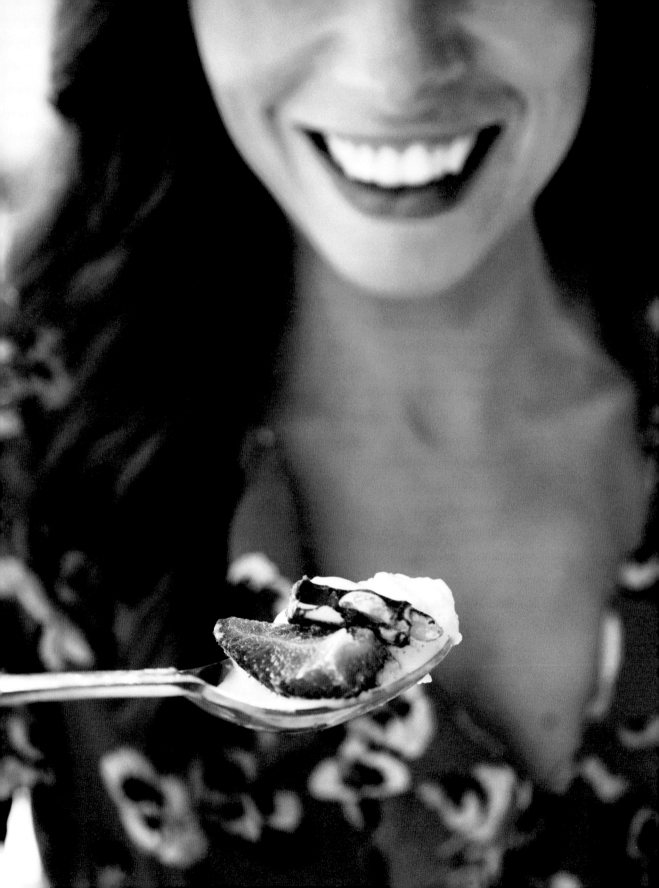

THE FEELGOOD GUIDE TO
SWEET TREATS

Just the right amount of sugar is yum-azing.
Here's how to do it right—and not overdo it

Any dessert you make yourself is going to make you feel better than a processed one that's full of artificial sugar, chemicals and preservatives, and has been sitting in the shop stockroom for the last few weeks. Home baking means you control the ingredients and know exactly what you're eating—so you appreciate every delicious mouthful. For feelgood baking, use organic ingredients and remember these smart swaps:

If making your own dessert isn't an option, think architectural:

be minimalist—the fewer ingredients, the better

deconstruct—eat the pie filling, not the pastry case. Scoop a spoonful of squirty cream to the side of your plate and enjoy the rest

When you're out and about, refer to the feelgood grid overleaf.

STOP THIS

white flour

all the sugar the recipe recommends

cooking chocolate

DO THIS

whole wheat flour

half the recommended sugar and a handful of fresh fruit

raw cacao powder

4 HEALTHY-IN-A-HURRY SWEET TREATS

1 **Banana ice cream:** unpeel and freeze a ripe banana. Blend until smooth or eat as is

2 **Dark chocolate:** make it 70% for all the antioxidants and not too much sugar

3 **Peanut popcorn:** top a bowl of air-popped corn with a spoon of melted PB

4 **Fruity fro-yo:** stir frozen berries into Greek yogurt, freeze and enjoy

TREAT YOURSELF AND FEEL GOOD

FEELS BAD	FEELS OK	FEELS GOOD
Ice cream		
Soft-serve vanilla ice cream is just unhealthy fat, chemically altered sugar, flavorings and powdered cream. A sickly and unsatisfying result	Quality vanilla ice cream contains real cream, sugar and egg and vanilla—just a few delicious ingredients	Organic ice cream—the most wholesome versions of those fabulous few ingredients
Cookies		
Cookies with a shelf life of several months and a huge list of unpronounceable ingredients. They are manufactured with exactly enough unsatisfying sugar to make you want to pig out on the whole package	A freshly baked cookie from a bakery—you've got natural ingredients and portion control	Biscotti or ginger snaps demand more chewing, so you can't wolf them down—you have to take time to appreciate these cookies properly
Chocolate		
Fake chocolate. You know, the kind with lots of sugar, bad fats and not enough cocoa to satisfy your chocolate cravings	Organic milk chocolate has better-quality ingredients, which means a small bar will satisfy you perfectly	Organic dark chocolate is the absolute best. A few squares of the stuff can even help regulate your stress hormone, cortisol [16]. Choose a bar with 70% cocoa and you'll get extra antioxidants and mouth-melting loveliness, too
Chocolate dessert		
Profiteroles—unsatisfying syrupy chocolate with a lot of trans-fat-tastic pastry	Chocolate mousse, because it's only got a few ingredients and one of them is "air"	Melted chocolate fondue with fresh fruit dippers. The most deliciously wrapped sweet
Cake		
Plastic-wrapped, processed sponge cake with ganache filling and heavy frosting: that's three different sugary textures, and one big crash waiting to happen	Cake from a coffee shop that looks like it was baked recently, and only has a slim layer of icing	Freshly baked, hand-made sponge cake filled with real cream and fresh strawberries. It has the least ingredients, and they're natural

FEELS BAD	FEELS OK	FEELS GOOD
Cheesecake		
Instead of fresh fruit, there's syrupy-looking jam on top—fake sugar is unsatisfying empty calories. This processed monstrosity has a long shelf life thanks to its enormous chemical content	Restaurant cheesecake with fresh fruit on top	Freshly baked cheesecake with an Italian twist. Using ricotta instead of standard cream cheese means you get more hunger-satisfying protein, so a slim slice quickly makes you feel full
Cakes		
Millionaire shortbread is three layers of sugar stacked on top of one another	Chocolate brownie with pecans and hazelnuts, as some of the sugar is replaced by delicious nutty protein that helps you know when you've had enough	Crepe with nuts and seeds for extra-satisfying protein, fiber and healthy fats
Apple pie		
Pastry has no redeeming features: it is the unhealthiest kind of fat. Usually there is more gelatinous sugar than actual apples within processed pies like this	Classic apple crumble—a little bit dull, but hearty, too	With an oaty crumble topping you get a good dose of tryptophan, an amino acid that boosts your "happy hormone" serotonin
Meringue		
Lemon meringue pie sounds virtuous, but its cookie base is usually made from trans-fat-packed cookies, and a lot of sugar is added to counteract the tartness of the lemon	Pavlova beats lemon meringue pie because it skips the cookie base and has real fruit, too	Eton Mess involves small chunks of meringue, which means less sugar mixed with your fresh strawberries and cream
Fruity desserts		
Jelly. It sounds light, but it's just sugar without any of fruit's natural fiber	Stewed fruit with custard. It's OK, but be aware that fruit is usually steeped in a liqueur or orange juice—that sweetness doesn't come out of thin air	Fresh fruit with a dollop of cream or melted chocolate. So simple, so good

The big screen can be a big pitfall—here's how to deal

Let's be brutal: you don't **need** to eat when watching a film. You're sitting down for 2 hours—this does not require extra energy. As if your ticket wasn't pricey enough, cinemas make a third of their profits from the concession stand. Here's how they try to trick you into buying bucket-loads of bad food:

The popcorn conspiracy

An exhaust pipe pumps air from the popcorn machine all over the theatre as the smell stimulates your appetite even when you've already eaten. We eat a third more popcorn from large containers, even when it's stale, because the scale of the snack dupes us into not realising when we're full [17].

More horrors: a large container of popcorn can contain up to 75% of your recommended daily amount of sodium and about 1,800 calories. That's roughly the same amount as six regular burgers. Six! Would you even dream of eating six burgers as a post-dinner snack? No, you would not.

The comparison trap

We optimistically try to weigh up and compare the feelgood benefits of, say, hotdogs to slushies. Save yourself the bother: they're both rubbish.

The veil of darkness

We automatically eat more when the lights go out—the disarming effect on our inhibitions is akin to being drunk. Mindful eating at the movies is a challenge. Your best bet for taking advantage of the darkness is to sneak in your own snacks. So sue us, Odeon.

For those nights when you really want to eat a little extra, pick a feelgood treat from this grid. They're all alternatives to typical cinema snacks that are easy to stash in your bag and bring out when the lights go down...

MOVIE NIGHT MUNCHIES

FEELS BAD	FEELS OK	FEELS GOOD
Popcorn		
Toffee popcorn—a sugar mountain. The fact that it expires in a year suggests how difficult it is for your body to digest	The smallest carton of movie theatre popcorn, either sweet or salty, shared with a friend	Air-popped corn made at home, with your own pinch of sugar or sea salt. Failing that, a single bag of supermarket popcorn, because this "small" is a fraction of the size of the cinema's "small" portion
Ice cream		
Several scoops of different-flavored ice cream with sugar sprinkles, fudge sauce and chocolate chips	Two scoops of ice cream with only one topping	Two scoops (or one small pot) of quality ice cream. Remember, the fewer ingredients, the better
Nachos		
A mountain of nachos with synthetic processed cheese that's been sitting under that heat lamp forever	One small, single-serving bag of MSG-dusted nachos	A small bag of quality pita chips—the only ingredients you need are corn, oil and salt
Sweets		
A sack of trail mix, with loads of different types of sugars and a stomach-churning sprinkle of bacteria, too	Sharing a bag of gummy sweets with a friend	Bringing your own normal single-serving package of sweets from the newsstand
Chocolate		
A family-sized grab bag, when there's just you in your "family"	Sharing a bag of lighter chocolate—think honeycomb instead of toffee—with a friend	Dark chocolate with 70% cocoa from your private stash—you probably won't find this delicacy in a cinema
Fizzy drinks		
A vat of soda from the post-mix machine	A can of soda—it may be sugary but it's portion-controlled	A bottle of sparkling water

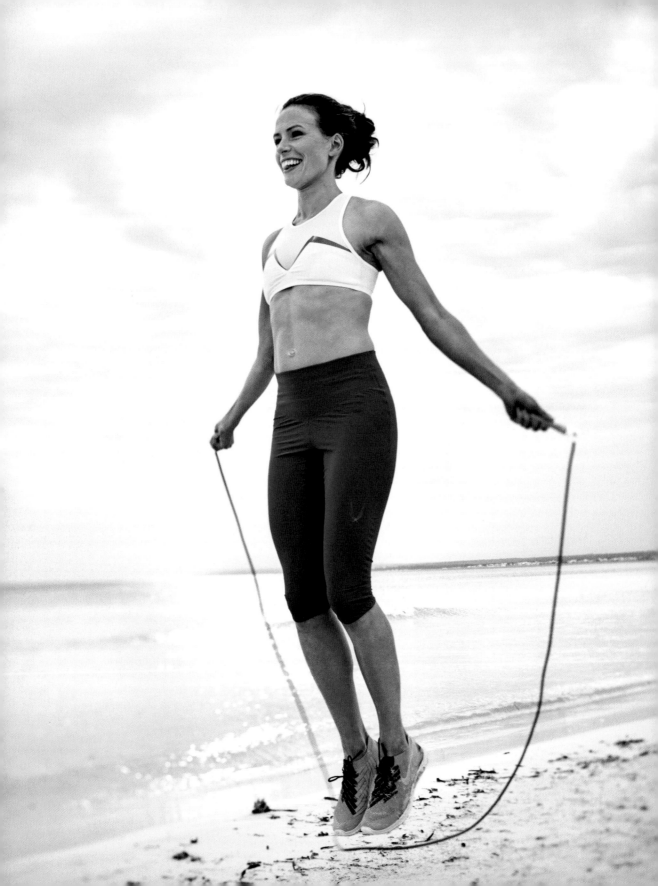

PART 3

MOVE

Find the right exercise for you, right now, and you've found the route to feeling better. In this section you'll discover how to up your energy, get fitter, strengthen your body and avoid pesky aches and pains. Oh, and you'll learn how much you can really get away with eating when you're in great shape (clue: it's a lot)

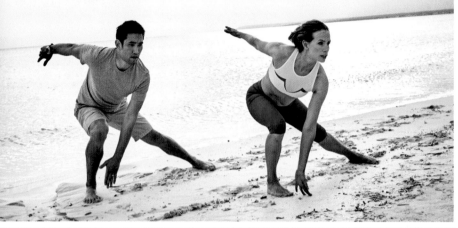

FIND YOUR PERSONAL WORKOUT PLAN

10

Say hello to the fitness routine that makes you feel so good you'll want to do it

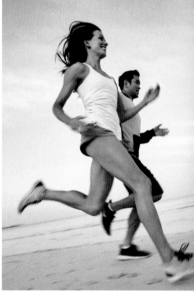

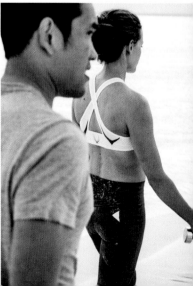

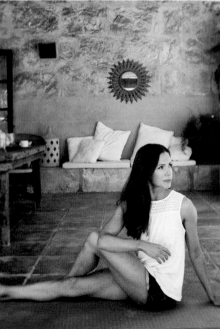

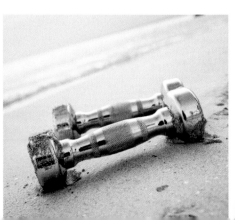

Exercise is about feeling good—looking your best is just the silver lining

In fact, flexing your body is a luxury. Don't believe it? Working out is scientifically proven to help you sleep, make you more productive, cut cravings and stimulate your "happy hormone", serotonin [1]. Lying on the sofa elbow-deep in a tub of ice cream does none of those things.

Unconvinced? Make a note of how uncomfortable and dissatisfied you feel after a lazy junk binge and compare it with the afterglow of an invigorating workout. It doesn't take long to realize which makes you feel better. And the high you get from exercise is far more sustainable.

Starting right now, we're going to change your relationship with exercise. The key to loving it is making the routine work for you. Happily, this personalized plan is:

Easy-going: tell yourself you can always stop. The key is to get going, because after the first few minutes, you won't want to give up.
Convenient: sometimes the hardest thing about exercise is getting out of the front door, so every workout in this book can be done in your own home, in your own time, without fancy equipment.
Do-able, yet effective: the feelgood workouts will ease you in gently yet you will sweat, so you work out at the right fitness level for your body.
Sustainable: these workouts will push you just enough to get results, but not so hard you'll want to give up.

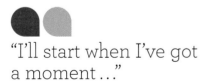

"I'll start when I've got a moment…"

Maybe work is crazy or you've got plans every weekend—don't worry, you can still find 1% of your day to fit an easy 15-minute workout into your life. The more overworked, tired or busy you feel, the more you need to take time to look after your body. Seriously: it's science. Bosses who don't make time for fitness feel stressed and are abusive to their staff, unlike managers who do [2]

> **Take 15 minutes to schedule your workouts for the week ahead—then you'll get them done**

FIND THE EXERCISE PLAN THAT TAKES YOU TO THE TOP

In the next three chapters, you'll find workout plans designed to zoom you up to the feelgood zone, even if you're at rock bottom right now. At each level, there is an explanation of exactly what to do and when to do it. Use this mood curve to find your starting point.

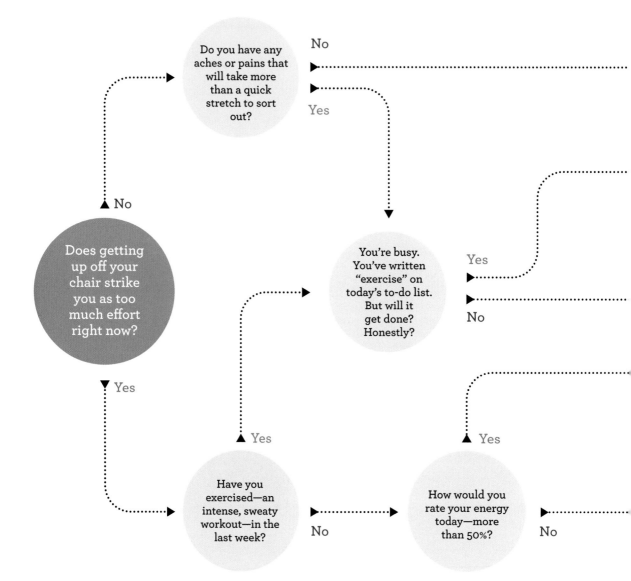

Do you have any aches or pains that will take more than a quick stretch to sort out?

No

Yes

No

Does getting up off your chair strike you as too much effort right now?

Yes

You're busy. You've written "exercise" on today's to-do list. But will it get done? Honestly?

Yes

No

Yes

Yes

Have you exercised—an intense, sweaty workout—in the last week?

No

How would you rate your energy today—more than 50%?

No

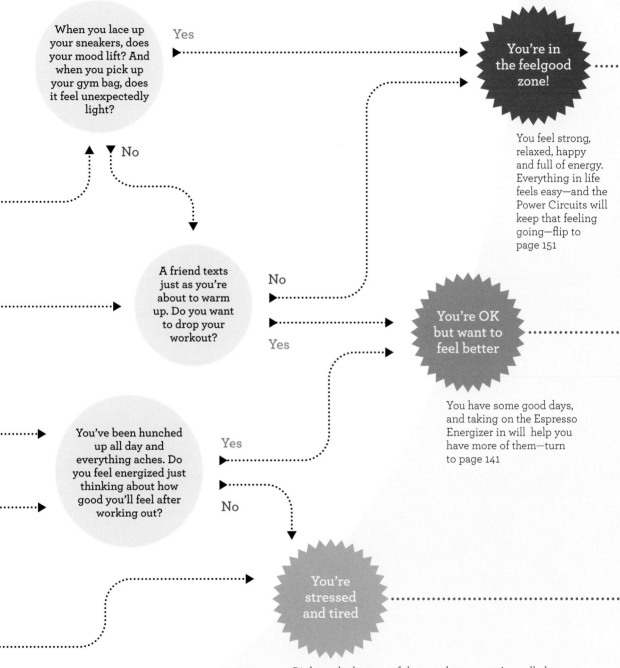

When you lace up your sneakers, does your mood lift? And when you pick up your gym bag, does it feel unexpectedly light?

Yes

No

You're in the feelgood zone!

You feel strong, relaxed, happy and full of energy. Everything in life feels easy—and the Power Circuits will keep that feeling going—flip to page 151

A friend texts just as you're about to warm up. Do you want to drop your workout?

No

Yes

You're OK but want to feel better

You have some good days, and taking on the Espresso Energizer in will help you have more of them—turn to page 141

You've been hunched up all day and everything aches. Do you feel energized just thinking about how good you'll feel after working out?

Yes

No

You're stressed and tired

Right at the bottom of the mood curve, you're really low on energy, everything feels like too much effort and you feel old before your time. The Anti-Aging plan will turn things around for you—start on page 131

HOW TO WANT TO EXERCISE
"Sloth on the sofa," you say? Here's your five-step plan for tuning in to what your body is *really* trying to tell you

STEP 1

Shush your lazy voice
Don't give your excuses airtime: have your yoga mat rolled out on your bedroom floor so you work out first thing, or pack your kit in your bag so you're ready to go at lunchtime. Treat the "noooo" voice in your head as you would an errant toddler. Politely but firmly get started. You know best.

STEP 2

Spot your tipping point
Your body might creak as you warm up, but every stretch releases tension and every movement makes oxygen flow a little faster. The more aware you are of the moment your mood tips from miserable to happy, the more intense it feels.

STEP 3

Make a power playlist
Gloria Estefan knew her stuff: the rhythm is gonna get you. Listening to music helps you run farther, cycle longer and swim faster—often without you noticing the extra effort [3]. Songs with 120–140 beats per minute make you perform best. You can download software that organizes your whole iTunes library by its bpm, but "Beat It" by Michael Jackson (139bpm) will get you started.

STEP 4

Exercise mindfully
"Switching on" muscles with your mind can make them tone up 35% faster [4]. Mindful exercise is a moment-by-moment awareness of what your body's doing. Observe how your abs engage when you lift a weight. Feel every muscle in your feet push up from the ground as you run. Pay attention to the fact that you're getting healthier and stronger with every movement—it's a double positive reinforcement. The more mindfully you work out, the more you get hooked on the sensation of exercise, not just the results.

STEP 5

Bottle your post-workout glow
As you shower, take a moment to absorb how much happier, calmer and better you feel about yourself now. The feelgood flush you get after exercise is what will keep you coming back for more.

When you sweat, everyone wins.

Take a moment to think about how people you care about will benefit from you being fitter, calmer, stronger. Perhaps it means you swoop your kids into your arms for more cuddles, or you take fewer sick days, or you've got more sex drive. Maybe it means you leave the office dead on time because you've blasted through everything you need to do, or you can quickly get ready for a night out because the first outfit you throw on actually looks great. Just 15 minutes of exercise improves your day—and everyone else's, too.

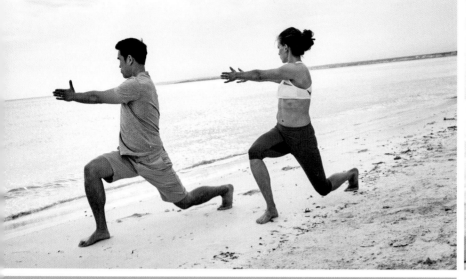

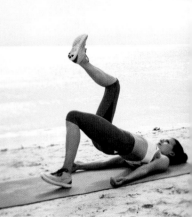

THE ANTI-AGING WORKOUT PLAN

11

Exercise gently to pick yourself up when you're stressed and tired

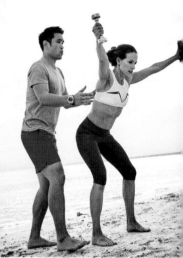

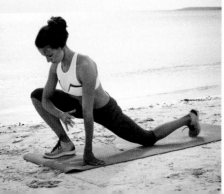

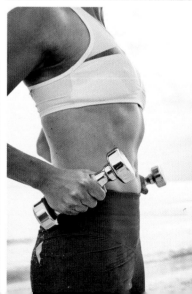

ANTI-AGING EXERCISE
When you feel lazy and you've got zero energy, this easy fitness plan will be kind to your body

One quick look at the plan (right) and you'll see it's the very reverse of gruelling. Focus on restoring and recharging and you'll soon feel like your old self—in fact, you'll feel like your younger self. Here's the plan:

Start with as little as 15 minutes of exercise, 4 days a week. Totally do-able. You don't have to buy a fancy outfit or go to the gym—you can do this workout in your underwear in the privacy of your own bedroom.

The Anti-Ager, a 15-minute body-weight circuit, will boost your energy and make you look and feel younger. The benefits start kicking in straight away, as movement stimulates serotonin, your natural feelgood neurotransmitter.

The Rest + Stretch duo will release stress and bodily tension. Wave bye-bye to the black cloud hanging over your head. You'll enjoy exercise. Yes, you will. Even if you snort with disbelief as you read this. At the weekend you'll treat yourself to whatever exercise you enjoy doing. Your cravings will wane, thanks to the 15-minute solution on page 137.

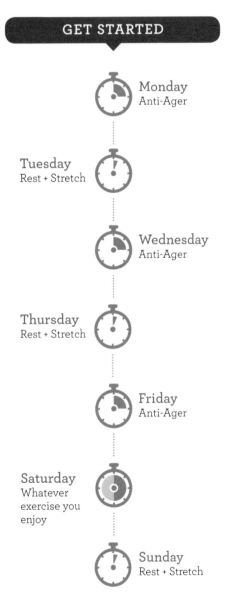

GET STARTED

Monday
Anti-Ager

Tuesday
Rest + Stretch

Wednesday
Anti-Ager

Thursday
Rest + Stretch

Friday
Anti-Ager

Saturday
Whatever exercise you enjoy

Sunday
Rest + Stretch

WARM-UP STRETCHES

Take one breath per movement; inhale through your nose and exhale through your mouth. Do each stretch five times each side

❶ Knee hugs

* Hug your left knee to your chest
* Keep your right leg flat
* Repeat x4, then switch

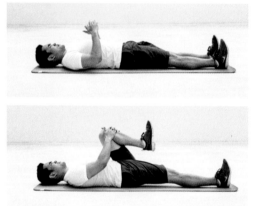

❷ Hamstring flicks

* Hold behind your knee
* Straighten your leg
* Repeat x4, then swap sides

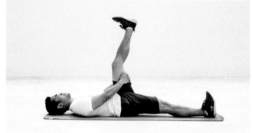
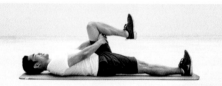

Struggling to get started?

Think of a time when you were calm in a crisis or said exactly the right thing. Feeling powerful can help make exercise seem easier. Recalling a scenario you handled well can actually make a heavy weight feel 20% lighter [1].

❸ Thread the needle

* Thread your left hand through to your
  right side to hover an inch above the floor
* Lift your hand above your left shoulder
  and look up. Feel your chest open
* Done 5? Repeat on your right

❹ Lunge stretch

* From a lunge position, place hands either
  side of your front foot
* Use your right elbow against your right knee
  to deepen the stretch
* Shoot your butt back to straighten your
  front leg and stretch the hamstring
* Do 4 more, then 5 on the other leg

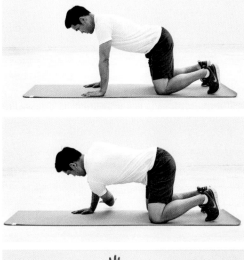

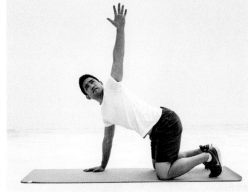

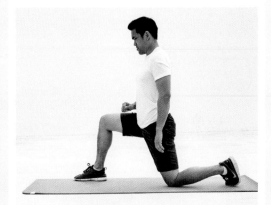

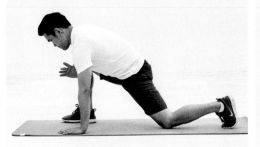

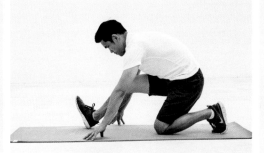

Go to thefeelgoodplan.com
to see the workout video

THE ANTI-AGER CIRCUIT

Perform the first 7 moves for 1 minute each, moving quickly from one to the next. Repeat. Then do the 60-second finisher. Go!

Need more motivation? Once you hit 30, not exercising is more of a health risk than smoking [2]. Happily, strength-training circuits like this one can reverse muscle aging by an incredible 6 years in just 10 weeks [3]. Want a youthful complexion too? Exercise releases myokines, protein messengers that help regenerate your skin by decades [4].

❶ Reverse lunge

* From standing take a big step back and lower your right knee
* Squeeze your left butt cheek and push through your heel to stand
* Alternate sides for 60 seconds

❷ T-bird

* Let your arms hang down and turn your thumbs out
* Raise your arms to create a T-shape
* Squeeze between your shoulder blades and keep your core engaged

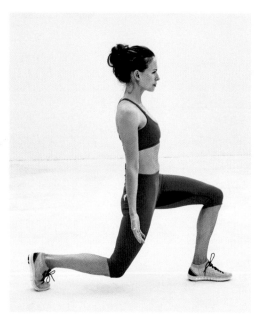

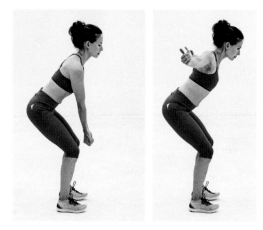

Yes, you've got time, the Anti-Ager is only 15 minutes—remember, that's just 1% of your day

❸ Squat salutation

* Drop into a half squat, keeping your arms level with your torso
* Shoot your hips forward and raise your arms to stand

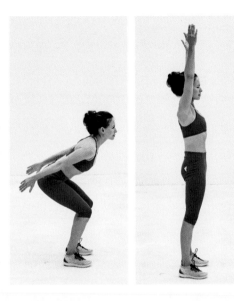

❹ Stairway to heaven

* Keep your head, hips and heels in one straight line
* Do a push-up, lowering slowly
* Squeeze between your shoulder blades and punch back up, fast

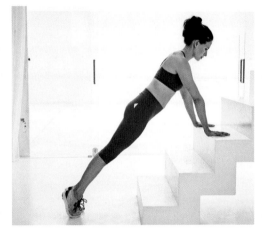

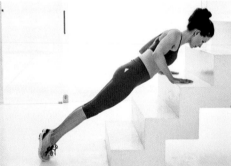

circuit continued overleaf >>>

❺ Step up

* Engage your right butt cheek, plant your right foot and step up
* Lift your left foot up, too
* Step down, then repeat on the left, alternating sides for 60 seconds

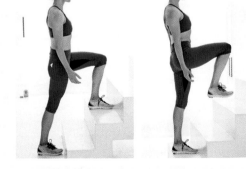

TIP — **Form is more important than speed**
It's OK to take a break if you can't do each move for a full minute. Just do as many as you can as well as you can, and gradually you'll notice you can do more and more.

❻ Single leg lowering

* Squeeze your naval towards your spine to engage your core
* Very slowly, swap the position of your legs
* Keep alternating for 1 minute

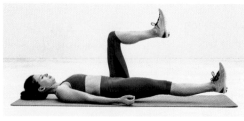

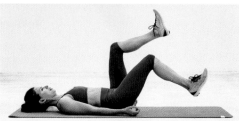

❼ Stork stance

* Easy peasy: raise your right knee to hip height
* Engage your abs to keep your spine straight
* Switch sides after 30 seconds

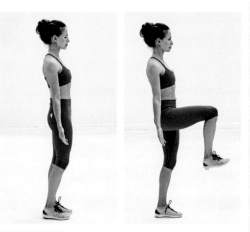

Repeat this circuit once more, then end with ...

The finisher: no-hands stand-up

* From lying down, stand up without using your hands or elbows
* Repeat for 1 minute
* Need motivation? The ease with which you can get up is closely linked to your chances of living longer [5]. So what you do in this minute could add years to your life

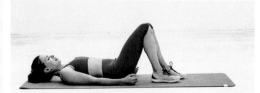

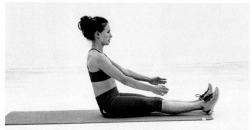

Exercise can reduce your genetic predisposition to weight gain by 40%—doesn't that make you feel good already? [6]

REST + STRETCH

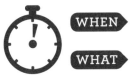

WHEN ▸ Tuesday, Thursday and Sunday

WHAT ▸ On rest days, use the warm-up stretches (pages 132–3) to "work in" to your body and tease away tension. The stretches are so gentle they can be done first thing in the morning, last thing at night or any time inbetween. The movement will relax you for the day or help you sleep—whatever your body needs at that time. You don't even need to wear gym attire—PJs will be just fine.

CRAVE-BUSTING WALK

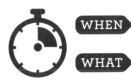

WHEN ▸ Every time cravings strike (so that'll be most days, then)

WHAT ▸ Stroll off your urge for a snack. Walking for 15 minutes can seriously reduce chocolate cravings by 50% [7]. Taking a walk means removing yourself from temptation while getting serotonin-boosting movement and daylight. Hello, happiness.

YOUR FREESTYLE WORKOUT

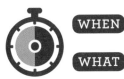

WHEN ▸ Saturday

WHAT ▸ Whatever activity you enjoy—golf, Pilates, cycling, running— it's the key to maxing the feelgood benefits. If you still dread the thought of exercise, get fit with a friend. As well as having someone to roll your eyes at and synchronize groans with, having a workout buddy adds a fun, competitive edge to your workout, whatever your level. Still not convinced? Exercising with a friend helps you lose more weight [8].

YOUR EXERCISE PROBLEMS SOLVED

"I feel "too fat" to exercise"

Even though the rational part of our brains knows that exercise will help us lose the weight that bothers us, sometimes we feel so negative about our size we don't feel up to moving at all. That gets us further away from feeling good: we find that we go down the mood curve.

Why do we self-sabotage like this? Because negativity makes us want to seal ourselves off from the world. This goes against the very nature of exercise, which makes our bodies open up, throw our shoulders back and stand tall.

What's more, when we're out of shape, exercise is harder work.

But if you're not happy with your body, then take the chance to do something about it. The Anti-Aging workout starts gently so you'll begin to get a feelgood buzz. Exercise is about far more than how we look; it's about realising what your amazing body is capable of. Getting fit will either give you a flat stomach or teach you to love the belly that you have.

"I've barely exercised since PE class'

Don't worry! Starting to work out now can reduce your risk of future illness by up to 45% [9].

"How can exercise be relaxing?'

Physical activity can help cut out the chatter in your head and keep you focused on the now, instead of worrying about things that may happen in the future, or that have happened in the past. If your attention wanders, bring your focus back to your breath. It helps you to stop grimacing and let oxygen do its peaceful feelgood flow.

"I haven't got dumbbells'

Use water bottles. The smaller weights you need for the Anti-Ager are easy to handle. As a guide, 1kg is 1 litre and 5 lb is, you guessed it, 2 litres.

"I can't be bothered today"

Just show up. No one ever regrets doing a workout, but you will regret not doing it.

"What's the point of strength training?'

Weight-training boosts your metabolism up to 30%, because having more lean muscle means you continue burning extra calories long after you've finished sweating. So you can have your cake, eat it and feel good about it, too. Perhaps you want to give up before you've finished the first minute. By the third, you'll feel ready to die. But after the fifth, the feelgood hormones have kicked in and you're having fun. Pay attention to what's going on in your head. Watch your brain closely, like a detective would study CCTV footage. Feel that buzz of pleasure. There you have it. Those are the endorphins. And the more exercise you do, the bigger that buzz will get. Oh, and you're officially in fat-burning mode now, too—there's another incentive to keep at it.

FEELING OK? LET'S GO UP A LEVEL

You're ready for the Espresso Energizer when...

- [ ] The Anti-Ager feels easy
- [ ] You no longer feel exhausted and achy
- [ ] You want more feelgood buzz
- [ ] You want to lose weight

Use these upgrades to propel your body up the mood curve:

❶ Reverse lunge

Hold 5 lb weights in each hand and curl them up to your shoulder with every lunge.

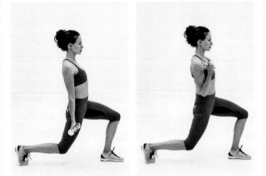

❷ T-bird

Hold 2 lb weights in each hand.

❸ Squat salutation

Squat lower—the sweet spot is when your thighs are parallel to the floor.

❹ Stairway to heaven

Push up from a lower step.

❺ Step-up

Choose a higher step, or hold weights in your hands.

❻ Single leg lowering

Extend your leg out lower to the floor and hold.

❼ Stork stance

Balance on an uneven surface like a pillow or rise up onto your toes.

The finisher: No-hands stand-up
Get up with your eyes closed.

Keep moving up with the Espresso Energizer workout plan, over the page.

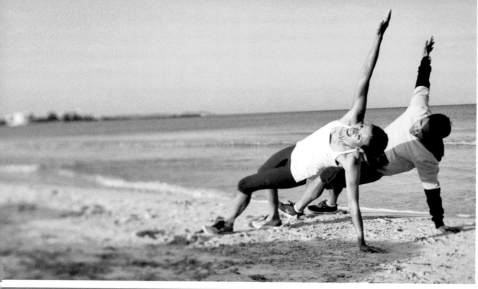

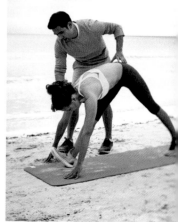

THE ESPRESSO ENERGIZER WORKOUT PLAN 12

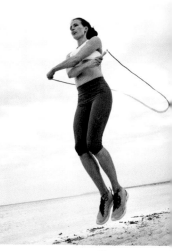

You could carry on doing what you're doing, but why not enjoy life more? This chapter is designed to arugula-launch you up to the feelgood zone

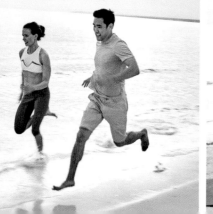

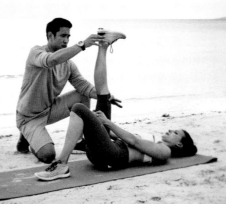

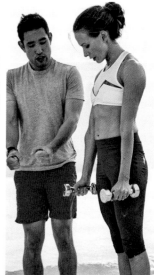

You have good days where you're bursting with energy. But there are several more bad days than you'd like, when you wish you'd stayed in bed. Let's change things...

This plan focuses on building strength, toning up and getting more energy into (and out of) your workouts. Here goes:

The Espresso Energizer strength circuit wakes up your energy, increases your metabolism and tones muscle; High-intensity sprintervals blast fat and build endurance; Low-intensity stretches de-stress and repair your body so you feel even better.

This triple whammy will take you to the top of the mood curve. Along the way, you'll notice you start eating and sleeping better, too.

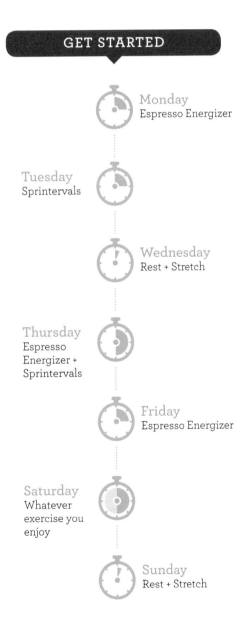

GET STARTED

Monday
Espresso Energizer

Tuesday
Sprintervals

Wednesday
Rest + Stretch

Thursday
Espresso
Energizer +
Sprintervals

Friday
Espresso Energizer

Saturday
Whatever
exercise you
enjoy

Sunday
Rest + Stretch

On Thursdays, choose whether you do your workouts back-to-back (take 3 minutes' rest between them) or do 15 minutes in the morning and 15 minutes at lunchtime

WARM-UP STRETCHES

Take one breath per movement: inhale through your nose and exhale through your mouth. Do each stretch five times each side

❶ Knee hugs

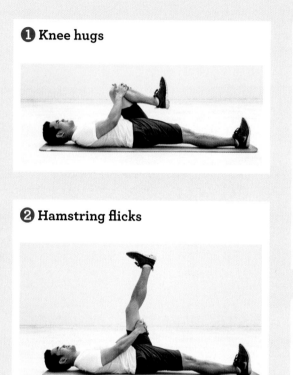

❷ Hamstring flicks

❸ Thread the needle

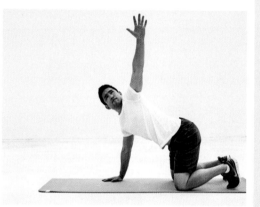

❹ Lunge stretch

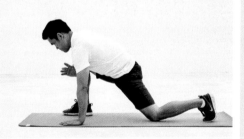

ESPRESSO ENERGIZER

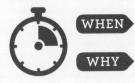

WHEN Monday, Thursday and Friday—and again whenever cravings strike

WHY This do-anywhere workout will wake up your brain, rev up your metabolism and deliver restorative oxygen to muscles that need it most. It gives you a similar adrenaline buzz to caffeine and an extra shot of feelgood serotonin, too. How's that for energising?

1 Pendulum lunge

* Step back with your right foot and lower your right knee
* Put your weight in your left heel and take a big step forwards with your right leg, so now your left knee hovers above the floor
* Repeat on the left leg, alternating for 1 minute

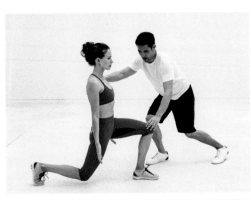

2 Kneeling push-ups

* Bend your elbows and lower your chest to the ground with control
* Punch up until the elbows are straight
* Remember to engage your abs and between your shoulder blades

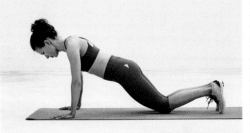

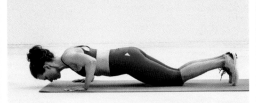

circuit continued overleaf >>>

❸ Back toner

* Drop into a shallow squat, with arms hanging down
* Holding a light weight in each hand, bend your arms and move your elbows in line with your ribcage
* Squeeze your abs to maintain a straight spine

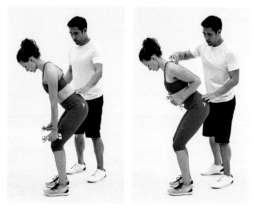

❺ Squats

* Hold a 5 lb weight up to your chest
* Push your bottom backwards, slowly lowering until your thighs are parallel to the floor
* Squeeze your butt and push through your heels to stand

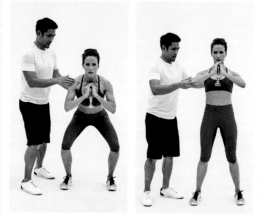

❹ Mountain climber

* Start in plank: head, hips and heels in one straight line
* Bring your left knee to your chest for 1 second
* Continue swapping legs for 1 minute

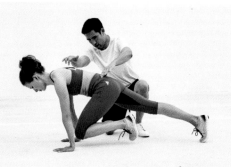

❻ Side plank

* Lift everything but your forearm and the side of your foot off the ground
* Keep your hips stacked and body straight
* After 30 seconds, switch sides

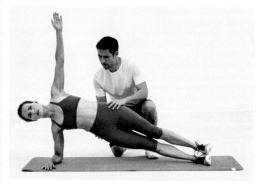

❼ Back extensions

* Lie face down and lift your head and arms 3 inches off the floor
* Hold for 10 seconds, then lower
* Repeat until your minute is up

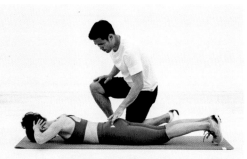

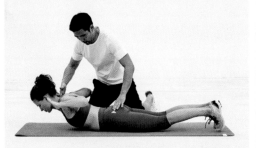

Run through that energising circuit once more from the top, then do 1 minute of . . .

The finisher: Box clever

* Sink into a half squat, fists at your armpits
* Sharply punch out your left arm, fist in line with your shoulder
* Fight the good fight for 1 minute, alternating arms and striking clean, firm punches

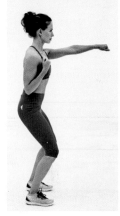

Check out thefeelgoodplan.com to see these moves in action

Got cravings? Save yourself from a snack attack

The strength-training circuit in this workout has been specially designed to save you from unhealthy cravings. You know from the Anti-Ager plan that walking can put the kibosh on cravings, but now you're fitter, your body will benefit from extra challenge.

Working out trains more than your muscles: it flexes your brain's willpower reserve, too. Just one workout acutely reduces snack cravings [1].

There's more: exercise actually changes the function and structure of the brain to strengthen self-control. Neurological scans show regular exercisers have more grey matter in the prefrontal cortex, which governs impulse control, focus, stress-management and self-awareness [2].

Next time you feel your willpower weaken, take action—literally—with this crave-cracking workout. You can do this routine in front of the TV, right on the craving battlefield, without any special equipment. Just one round is enough to take the edge off.

SPRINTERVALS

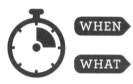

WHEN ▸ Tuesday and Thursday

WHAT ▸ A gentle 3-minute run at 70% effort, followed by 15 seconds sprinting all out. Repeat these speed intervals for 15 minutes—that's four rounds. You'll get results fastest if you change up your cardio every week. Alternate running with skipping, spinning, rowing, swimming or blasts on the cross-trainer. Whatever exercise you do, maintain the 3 minutes steady/15 seconds sprinting ratio.

REST + STRETCH

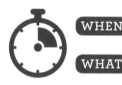

WHEN ▸ Wednesday and Sunday

WHAT ▸ Give yourself a break! But it's not all about lying on the sofa. The slow, restorative stretches in the warm-up stretches (page 142) get your blood flowing and repair your muscles, so you're able to handle high-intensity training without wanting to spend the rest of the week in a wheelchair.

YOUR FREESTYLE WORKOUT

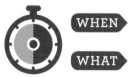

WHEN ▸ Saturday

WHAT ▸ Try dynamic yoga, kickboxing or a reformer pilates class. Your freestyle session is a prime opportunity to listen to your body—do you want to stretch out with ballet, escape with a long run or release tension leaping around the tennis court? You don't always have to push yourself physically; just do whatever feels right.

GO UP TO THE FEELGOOD ZONE

Use the upgrades below to make the Espresso Energizer more challenging, and you'll soon go up to the feelgood zone. Start by doing the upgrades for the first 15 seconds, then switch back to the regular version on pages 143–5

❶ Pendulum lunge

Curl a pair of light weights up to your shoulders and push overhead as you hold every lunge.

❷ Kneeling push-ups

Time for full push-ups: toes are on the floor and head, hips and heels are in one straight line.

❸ Back toner

Lift a heavier weight.

❹ Mountain climber

Sprint.

❺ Squats

Jump, and squat immediately as you land.

❻ Side plank

Raise your top leg to create a star shape.

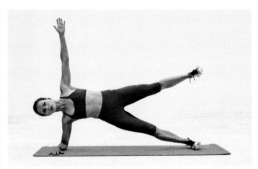

❼ Back extensions

Lift your limbs another 2–3 in.

The finisher: Box clever

Hold a 5 lb weight in each hand.

SPEED UP YOUR SPRINTERVALS

As you get fitter, reduce the length of your gentle run by 15 seconds with every workout until you're fit enough to sprint 15 seconds on/15 seconds off. Relax, you never need repeat the intervals for more than 15 minutes.

When that gets easy (it will, promise!), throw an extra set of speed intervals into your schedule, so on Monday you do sprintervals after your strength training.

Stay at the top of your mood curve with the Power Circuits on page 150

Go back to the Anti-Ager for a week if . . .

When three or more of these symptoms feel familiar, take things easy:

* You wake up tired.
* All day long, your energy is low.
* Sex? No, thank you.
* You've got constant aches and pains you can't stretch out.
* You feel like your body is working overtime.
* Getting through the day on anything less than three coffees feels impossible.
* You crave salty, fatty and sweet foods— not from physical hunger, but to find an emotional fullness.
* You want a glass of wine, but when you drink it you feel down, not relaxed.

How long until you see results?
Give yourself 2 weeks to tone your muscles, then you'll start shedding fat.

Will weights turn you into the Incredible Hulk?

In a word: no. Biology dictates that women don't naturally have the testosterone to reach Incredible Hulk dimensions. Bulking up requires testosterone, a huge calorie surplus and very heavy weights. That's not what you're doing: you're just using light dumbbells to burn residual body fat. You're not lifting anything too heavy—you're lifting just enough weight to elicit a response.

We can all benefit from building more lean muscle. It's the magic ingredient that tones your body and boosts your metabolism (so you burn more calories when you're doing important stuff like watching TV). Having more lean muscle also improves your heart, bone and joint health.

WHAT WEIGHTS SHOULD YOU USE?
Weights are supposed to be challenging, but never use anything that you can't lift at least fifteen times with perfect form. For the Espresso Energizer, start with 5 lb in each hand and work up to 6 lb or 10 lb.

If running makes your joints ache, choose a cardio that's less high-impact. Swimming, spinning or using a cross-trainer are great alternatives.

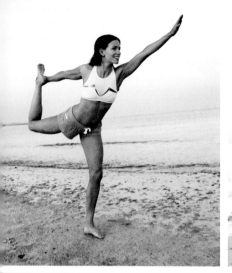

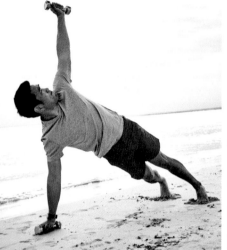

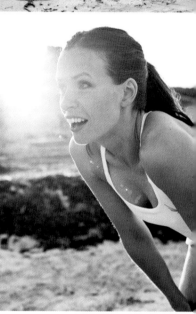

POWER CIRCUITS 13

You're fitter, faster and firmer now. To keep your body on an upward trajectory, simply crank the sweat-o-meter up to the next level

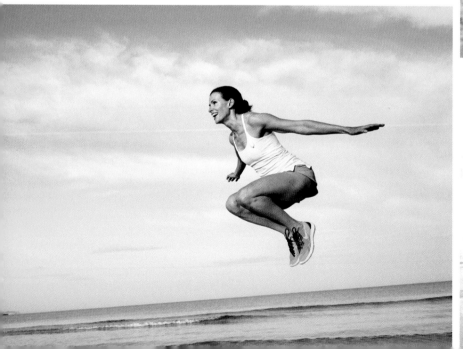

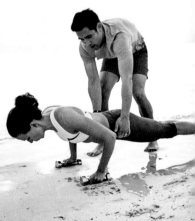

The workouts in this chapter are designed to keep you fit and energized, flying through the feelgood zone. Here goes:

You've got two new 15-minute Power Circuits. These workouts not only target-tone your bottom, legs, stomach and arms, but also give you more freedom food-wise. Oh, and the circuits will help relieve stress, zap back pain and smooth cellulite, too, making your life all-around easier;

Your sprintervals are still only 15 minutes but they get more intense, thanks to the fact that you're so much stronger now;

You're fitter now, so you're in prime condition to take on a race, like that triathlon you've had your eye on;

Your rest days can be more active, which means more fun. You're welcome.

This four-point plan will shoot your feelgood buzz to the sky. But as you go, keep checking in with your body so you're getting the exercise you need, without pushing yourself too far. Remember, your focus is on feeling good: you never need to beast yourself to look your best.

The trickier you find an exercise, the more you need to do it. Why? When you strengthen areas of weakness, your body is at optimum balance.

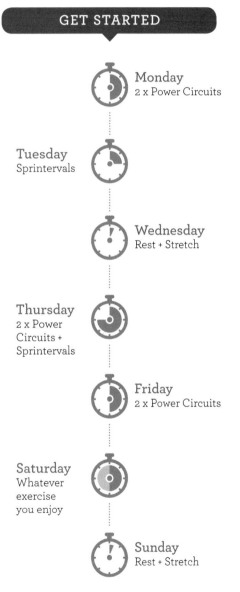

GET STARTED

Monday
2 x Power Circuits

Tuesday
Sprintervals

Wednesday
Rest + Stretch

Thursday
2 x Power Circuits + Sprintervals

Friday
2 x Power Circuits

Saturday
Whatever exercise you enjoy

Sunday
Rest + Stretch

How to fit fitness into your week

OK, it seems like a lot of exercise, but you can shimmy it into your schedule with little effort. Every workout can be broken down into 15-minute blocks—remember, that's just 1% of your day. So even when life feels hectic, you can enjoy this vital time for yourself. Use this guide to help you make it work.

MONDAY AND FRIDAY

2 x Power Circuits
Option 1: Break them down
Break the two workouts down so you do one in the morning and one at lunchtime or in the evening.
Option 2: Mix them up
Do the two circuits one after the other, with 3 minutes' rest between them. Get your breath back with a gentle walk (or flop on the floor—you choose).

THURSDAY

2 x Power Circuits + Sprintervals
Option 1: Break them down
Break the three workouts down so you do one in the morning, one at lunchtime and one in the evening.
Option 2: Mix them up
Sandwich the sprintervals between the Power Circuits, with 3 minutes' rest between each circuit.

WARM-UP STRETCHES

Before you start your workout, warm up with these moves. Think one breath per movement, inhaling through your nose and exhaling through your mouth. Do each stretch five times on each side

❶ Knee hugs

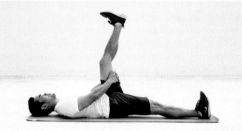

❷ Hamstring flicks

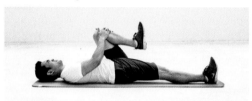

❸ Thread the needle

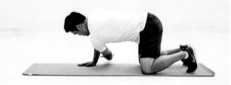

❹ Lunge stretch

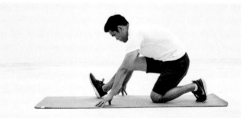

POWER CIRCUITS

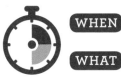

WHEN Monday, Thursday and Friday

WHAT Like strawberries and cream or Batman and Robin, some things are just better together. These two 15-minute circuits are designed around power couples: legs and butt and abs and arms. Do them back to back or break them down to snack-size portions—your choice.

LEGS AND BUTT:
the "see you later cellulite, hello feast" power couple

WHY Your legs and bottom are home to your biggest muscles, which make them fat-burning furnaces. In other words, nailing this workout gives you the freedom to indulge. As for cellulite, the weights in this circuit target-tone your leg and buttock muscles to make lumps and buttps less visible, while the boost to your circulation helps cleanse your lymphatic system, too.

WHAT Each round is 1 minute. Perform moves 1–4 twice, then do moves 5–7 twice, then complete the finisher.

ARMS AND ABS:
the "bye stress, hello easy life" power couple

WHY Firm abs can free you from back pain and aching knees [1], while toned arms can mean no more knotted shoulders, so you feel less stressed. As if that doesn't make life feel easy enough, having a flat stomach and toned arms makes most outfits look effortlessly good.

WHAT Each round is 1 minute. Perform moves 1–4 twice, then do moves 5–7 twice, then complete the finisher.

LEGS AND BUTT POWER CIRCUIT

❶ Dumbbell step-up

* Holding a weight in each hand, plant your right foot and step up
* Raise your left foot too
* Step down, then repeat on the left, alternating sides for 60 seconds

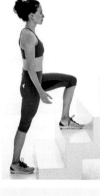

❷ Butt-lift deadlift

* Push your bottom backwards until your weights are level with your shins
* Keep your spine and arms straight
* Drive your hips forwards to stand

❸ Explode

* From a shallow squat, jump up
* Land softly, pushing your butt back into a squat

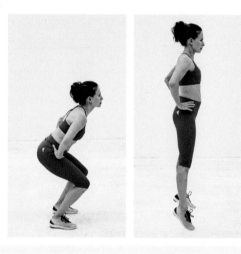

❹ Simple standing knee hug

* Raise your right knee to hip height
* Hold for 30 seconds, then switch sides

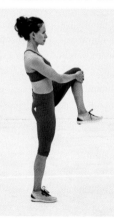

Repeat 1–4, then continue with ...

❺ Lateral lunge

* With a weight in each hand, hold the dumbbells either side of your bent right knee
* Balance 80% of your weight in your right heel
* Step to the center and repeat on your left

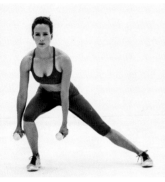

❼ Lunge jump

* Start in a lunge position
* Jump up and switch legs

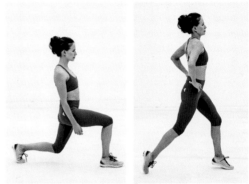

Repeat 5–7, then end with . . .

❻ Single leg squat

* Raise your right leg an inch off the floor
* Slowly squat on your left leg
* Alternate for 1 minute

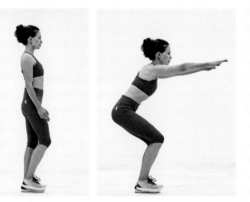

The finisher: Marching hip raise

* Squeeze your butt to float your hips up
* Tighten your right butt cheek and raise your left thigh to 45°
* Keep your hips high and lower with control. Switch legs for 1 minute

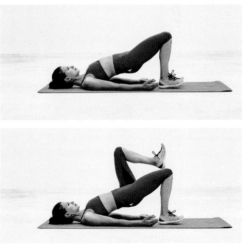

ARMS AND ABS POWER CIRCUIT

❶ Weighted push-up

* Start in plank position with a weight in each hand
* Lower your chest to the ground and press up
* At the top of your push-up, pull your left elbow into a row. Push up again, then row right.

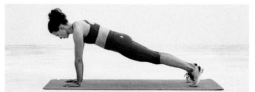

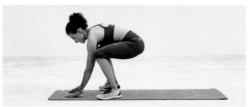

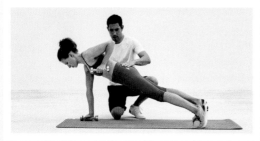

❷ Curl and press

* Start with arms hanging directly down and a weight in each hand
* Curl the weights to your shoulders
* Press the weights overhead, then lower down and repeat

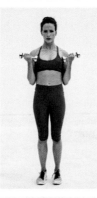

❸ Burpees

* From plank position jump both feet towards your chest
* Leap up to stand
* Plant your hands and jump back to plank

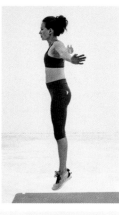

Repeat 1–4, then continue with . . .

❹ Corset plank sweep

* Start in side plank and extend your left arm overhead
* Lock your eyes on your hand as you slowly sweep it towards your right ribs
* Repeat for 30 seconds, then change sides

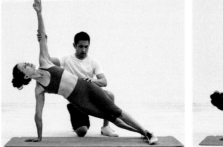

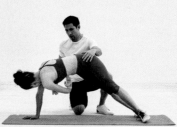

❺ Sideways raise with pulse

* With a weight in each hand, raise your arms to shoulder height
* Keep your arms straight and shoulders pulled down your back
* Pulse your hands an inch backwards 3 times, then lower and repeat

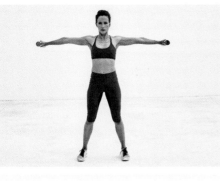

❻ High/low plank

* Start in plank, palms down
* Place your left elbow on the floor, then the right
* Push up to start position, then switch so you do the right elbow first

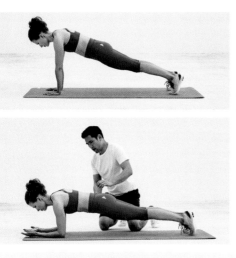

❼ Abs-olutely effective leg lowering

* Start with your knees at right angles
* Keeping abs squeezed tight, slowly straighten your legs
* Hold your legs out for 25 seconds, then rest for 5. Repeat
* The lower your legs hover above the floor, the more challenging this exercise is

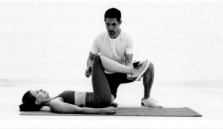

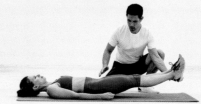

Repeat 5–7, then end with . . .

The finisher: Torpedo

* Looking at your mat, raise your head, chest and arms
* Push your hips into the floor and squeeze your naval in
* Hold for 25 seconds, then lower for 5 and repeat

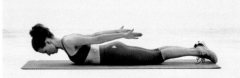

SPRINTERVALS

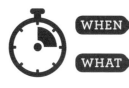

WHEN ▶ Tuesday and Thursday

WHAT ▶ Run at an easy pace for 2 minutes, then sprint all-out for 30 seconds. On an effort scale of one to ten, you're aiming for a nine. Repeat the interval for 15 minutes: that's six rounds.

REST + STRETCH

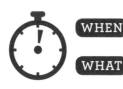

WHEN ▶ Wednesday and Sunday

WHAT ▶ You can be more active on rest days now you're fitter. As well as soothing your hard-working muscles with the restorative warm-up stretches (page 152), you might enjoy getting outside for a bike ride or just taking the dog for a big long walk. Save your can of whoopass for Saturday's freestyle session.

FREESTYLE WORKOUT

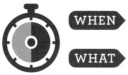

WHEN ▶ Saturday

WHAT ▶ Seeing as you're practically an Olympian now, consider trying a new sport. On top of the physical challenge, discovering new activities is scientifically proven to make you happier [2]. Having a strong core makes you a better runner, so consider taking on a race. Power training puts you in prime condition for muddy obstacle courses and adrenaline-infused ski vacations. And all those burpees mean sun salutations in dynamic yoga are a breeze.

STAY IN THE FEELGOOD ZONE— AND OFF THE PLATEAU

To keep your body responding to exercise, make one tiny upgrade to each workout: add two pounds to your normal weights or sprint for an extra five seconds. It pays to mix up your cardio, too: swap running for cardio like spinning, rowing or swimming.

Afterwards, listen to your body—was the workout more difficult? Do your muscles feel noticeably sorer, or are you tired out? If it was easy, add another change to your next workout, too. It usually takes 2 to 4 weeks to lift your body up off the plateau, so stick at it and don't be discouraged.

How was it for you?

Too easy	*Too tough*
Increase your weights	Lift lighter weights
Broaden your range of movement, so go lower on push-ups	Do less repetitions so you've got a break between each 1-minute set
Speed up, so you do more moves in every minute	Slow down. It's OK to pause between each rep

Trust your body to tell you when you need a break. If you're in pain, rest up. If you feel sore doing normal activities like climbing the stairs, but you don't want to miss a workout, go back to the Espresso Energizer circuit as it will stop you feeling so tired.

The truth about exercise and food

The fitter you are, the more you can get away with eating whatever you like, while staying in amazing shape and feeling great. Pompous much? Hell, yes

Here's a happy fact: you can be pretty liberal with what you eat after an intense workout like 45 minutes of Power Circuits and Sprintervals.

Ideally you'll fill your body with nourishing food like a chicken stir-fry, poached eggs or a protein shake, to firm your muscles, but we don't always like eating the healthiest thing on the menu. So on those occasions when you want to eat pizza, fries or whatever the hell you like, negate the damage by tucking in an hour or two after your Power Circuits + Sprintervals sandwich. That gives you enough time to shower and glide into your favorite restaurant guilt-free. Your food is absorbed instantly as your body needs the energy to repair muscle.

CRACK THE COFFEE CONUNDRUM

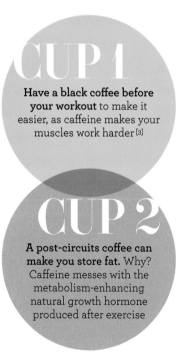

CUP 1

Have a black coffee before your workout to make it easier, as caffeine makes your muscles work harder [3]

CUP 2

A post-circuits coffee can make you store fat. Why? Caffeine messes with the metabolism-enhancing natural growth hormone produced after exercise

Intense interval workouts, like your Power Circuits + Sprintervals sandwich, can actually make you less hungry, as the exercise lowers your appetite-stimulating hormone, ghrelin [4].

It's OK to skive (sometimes) Well, there are five words you never expected to see in a fitness book

So, you went out instead of working out like you planned. Relax. This is only one day out of seven, so you have plenty of time another day to train. And you don't have to miss exercise completely—take a walk, do twenty squats while you wait for the kettle to boil, or just do the warm-up stretches (page 152) in front of the TV.

Missing a workout isn't the worst thing you can do. The worst thing you can do is to punish your body for playing hooky by bingeing on cookies. Or bingeing on anything, for that matter. Be especially mindful of what you eat on impromptu rest days: now, more than ever, you need nourishing food, not junk that will exhaust your tired body.

Occasionally, you might miss two or three workouts in a row. Cut yourself some slack if you get sick or if all hell breaks loose at work. But if gym-dodging becomes a trend, ask yourself what's going on. Are you not feeling a post-workout buzz? Is your exercise routine too difficult, or so easy it's ineffective? Figure out what's getting in the way and make the necessary adjustments.

Sometimes when we're tired, we forget that exercise gives us energy. Start gently—just warm up with the stretch sequence—and within a few mellow minutes you'll feel the boost that comes from more oxygen flowing to your brain and muscles. Then your serotonin activates, too, and your yawns are history.

If you hate exercise, stop it. Seriously. Give yourself a break for a week or two. This book is all about feeling good, remember? Focus on eating well and taking plenty of time to rest as this will balance your hormones and strengthen your body. When you're ready, pick your point on the mood curve (page 126) and start over. Working out because you want to, not because you **have** to, is a sure-fire way to bring on the feelgood glow.

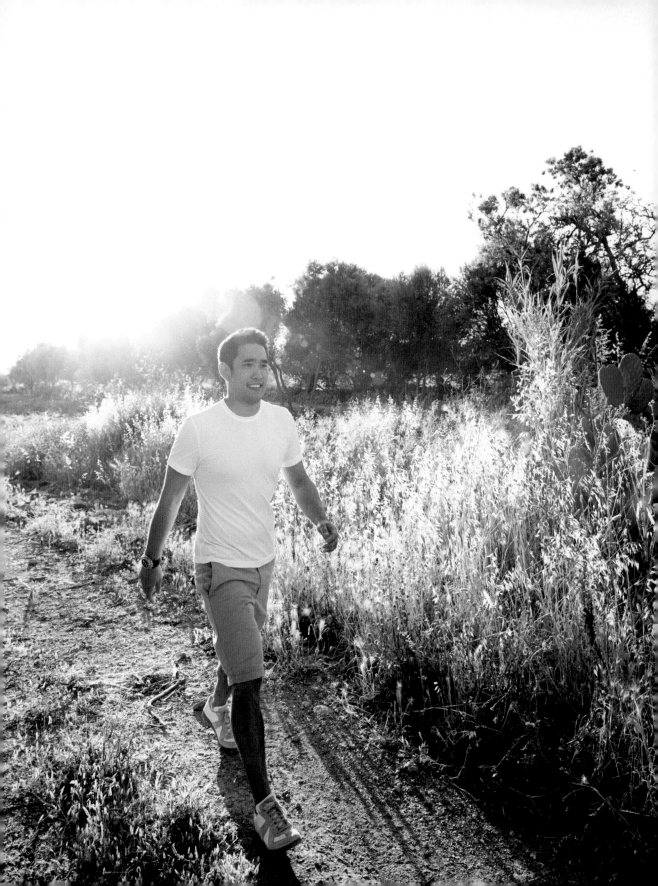

PART 4
RELAX

Everything you ever wanted to know about feeling less stressed, but were too exhausted to ask. This section will give you de-stressing strategies that help you sleep, see you through your working day, and make your me-time more meaningful. Because when you feel relaxed and happy, you naturally stay in great shape

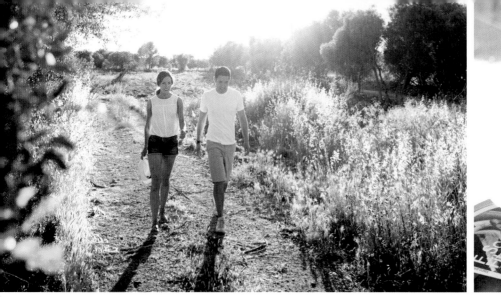

STOP WITH THE GO-GO-GO

14

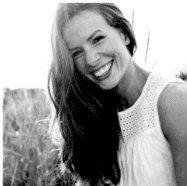

Why do you lose weight and get gorgeous skin on vacation without even trying? Because relaxation is essential to feeling and looking good

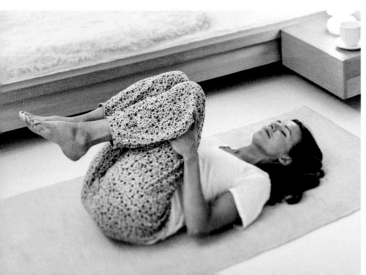

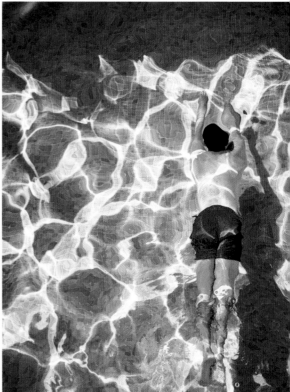

Sugar and alcohol are nothing compared to stress. The most harmful toxin of them all, stress can make you feel worse than any hangover.

In fact, left untreated, stress spreads faster than a yawn at an insomnia convention. We get impatient with our loved ones. We're edgy with people who try to help us. We sabotage our good intentions. We choose the quick and easy way out, then end up more frazzled than we started.

That's when we need to take a step back and focus on what's going on inside. Relaxing sets up a feelgood loop: it gives us the energy to make positive changes that give us even more energy. It's worth appreciating that stress happens when we're unhappy with how things are. It is your body's way of pushing you to make a positive change, so use it to your advantage.

You can't completely eliminate stress from your life. But you can learn healthy coping strategies that make difficult times less turbulent, help you take everything in your stride and make you happy to be *you* again. The road to recovery starts right here.

 Take a minimum of 15 minutes me-time daily. Phone your best friend. Dance to the radio. Have sex. Do whatever makes you happy

66% of us feel stressed before we even get out of bed [1]

CHECK IN WITH YOUR MOOD CURVE TO SAY GOODBYE TO STRESS

It's called "resting up" for a reason: because rest is what will lift your mood. Take a moment to see where you are today and find out how you could feel even better

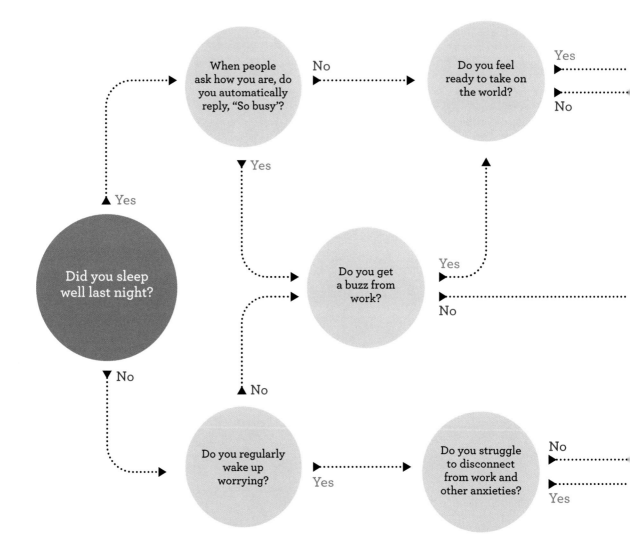

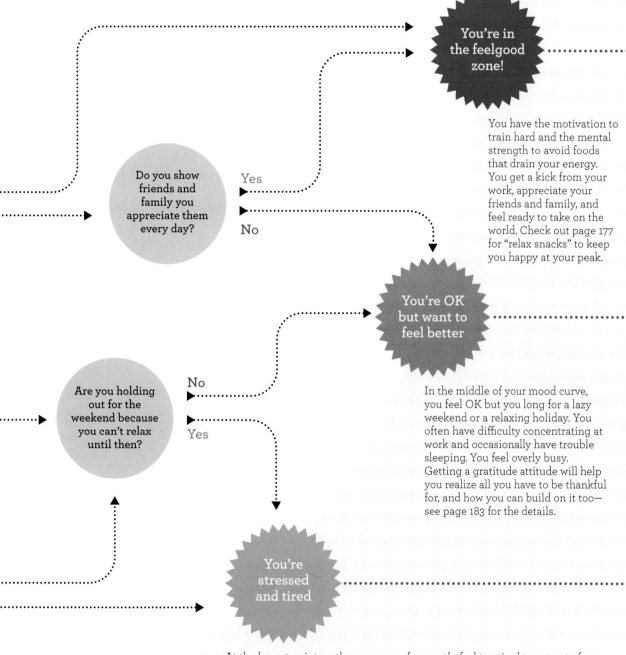

You're in the feelgood zone!

You have the motivation to train hard and the mental strength to avoid foods that drain your energy. You get a kick from your work, appreciate your friends and family, and feel ready to take on the world. Check out page 177 for "relax snacks" to keep you happy at your peak.

Do you show friends and family you appreciate them every day?

Yes

No

You're OK but want to feel better

In the middle of your mood curve, you feel OK but you long for a lazy weekend or a relaxing holiday. You often have difficulty concentrating at work and occasionally have trouble sleeping. You feel overly busy. Getting a gratitude attitude will help you realize all you have to be thankful for, and how you can build on it too—see page 183 for the details.

Are you holding out for the weekend because you can't relax until then?

No

Yes

You're stressed and tired

At the lowest point on the curve, you frequently feel too tired to get out of bed, yet you can't disconnect. You barely have time for the people you care most about. You wish you could call in sick and often wake at night worrying about work. This section will help you rediscover your ability to concentrate calmly, and show you the stretches that can help you sleep (page 182).

SEVEN SHORTCUTS TO A LESS STRESSED LIFE

1 **Forget perfect. It's better to feel good**
There's no such thing as perfect. But an insidious perfectionist streak can feel all too real. It pushes you to set unrealistic goals that make you feel like you're perpetually struggling to keep up. Curb your perfectionism by giving yourself a deadline and doing your best until that time is done. Has the world ended? No. Are you giving yourself room to breathe? Yes. Do you feel a little better already? Hope so.

2 **Stressed about being stressed?**
Instead of being hard on yourself, go easy on yourself. You're doing OK. You're reading this book, right now. You're on your way up.

3 **A blast of exercise will reduce anxiety**
Studies show that just 10 minutes does the trick; we find 15 minutes helps us feel happier and more focused [2]. Your workout doesn't have to be sweaty if you're dressed up for a big meeting—the Anti-Ager (page 134) or just a quick stroll calms your nerves.

4 **Achoo-mmmmm!**
Meditation is well-known for its ability to calm the mind, but can also boost your immune system so you're less likely to catch a cold, too [3].

5 **If you still haven't found what you're looking for, let go**
Analyzing a problem inside out can make you feel more frustrated than when you started. Sit back and let the answer come to you. The "aha" moment will bring your solution.

6 **Focus on what feels good**
Being happy isn't about avoiding stress completely (sorry, that's impossible); it's about paying attention to the good things in your life.

7 **When everything is too much**
In times of acute stress, take time out to let your emotions run their course. Don't worry about food or your exercise plan: rest is what you need to get through this difficult time. When your troubles aren't so all-consuming you'll go back to a healthier life: start with a daily walk and cooking yourself a nourishing dinner.

If stress goes straight to your stomach

This abdominal massage will help release tight muscles in your abdomen and diaphragm, which help digestion and reduce cramps. Here's what to do:

* Lie down and press your fingertips gently into the right side of your stomach, by your pelvic bone.
* Rub in a light circular motion up to your ribs, over to your left side, down to your left pelvic bone and back to your starting point.
* Repeat this clockwise motion, slowly increasing the pressure, for 5 minutes or until your bloating subsides.

The less stressed you are, the less you have to feel stressed about

Jokes are funnier, colors seem brighter, people seem kinder. You can live life to the full: enjoying cocktail hour or ordering a side of fries has negligible negative impact on your body, and indulging in a few treats doesn't mess up your head either. You find more pleasure from simple things and appreciate how lucky you are to be you.

Relax your way to a flatter stomach today

When we feel stressed, we burn over 100 fewer calories after eating [4]. What's more, fat cells in your midriff have four times the cortisol receptors of other fat cells, so when you're stressed out, cortisol binds to those cells and you store more fat. When you're chilled, you're effortlessly slimmer.

Wiggle away stress with a tennis ball

Knotted muscles and tight spots are physical pockets of stress in your body. Grab a tennis ball to bounce back into shape

A humble tennis ball is better used as foam roller: it helps increase circulation, mobilize muscles and release pain-relieving endorphins. Do this DIY massage after every workout for a speedy recovery. Inhale and exhale deeply three times—at least—for each area of tension you're working on. What aches today?

Your shoulders Hold the ball against the wall with the area inside your shoulder blade. Now, gently, shimmy on it until you feel tension ease off.

Your back So easy: put the ball on the wall and push your back into it. Roll up and down to soothe the overworked muscles each side of your spine (not on your actual bones). You could duct-tape two balls together to massage both sides of your back simultaneously.

Your hips Flip onto your front and place the ball at the inside of your right hip, right at the top of your thigh. Rest your body weight onto the ball to release the tight knot of muscle. This massage works wonders if you spend a lot of your day sitting at a computer or driving.

Your butt Sit your right butt cheek onto the ball. Bend your left knee and hook your right ankle over it to sink into the stretch and get the ball massaging deep into pain HQ. After 30 seconds, work on your right buttock.

Your legs Your legs appreciate being massaged from all angles:
Quads: Lie flat on the floor with the ball beneath your right thigh and repeat the same gentle wiggling action for 30 seconds on either leg.
IT bands: Lie on your side and use a long, sweeping motion to help the ball roll away tension from your outer thigh.
Hamstrings: Sit with the ball under your right thigh and push your weight down, letting gravity help locate and loosen any tender spots. Switch sides after 30 seconds.
Calves: Rest the back of your lower leg on the ball, pressing down for a deeper massage. Switch sides.

Your feet Hold a wall for balance then step onto the ball with your bare right foot. Gently rock backwards and forwards along the arch, where reflexology points are ripe, then repeat on your left foot. This is a great one to do before bed.

How often do you feel good when you're at work? Probably not enough.

Work stress ricochets from Mondays into the rest of our lives: it can make us distracted and unable to sleep, it drives us to overeat and gives us less time to exercise. When you're hit by these three factors simultaneously, your mood will sink down the curve.

Your job has a huge impact on your body: stress cuts through our lives like a machete, leaving us vulnerable to obesity, depression and other serious diseases [1]. Work-related tension even damages DNA in our cells—left unchecked, stress doesn't just make us feel old, it actually ages us [2].

In this chapter, you'll discover practical wellbeing strategies to stop being drained by your job, to sidestep stress-eating, and to help you switch off at the end of the day. Who knows, you might even start enjoying your work.

The new shape of success

"I'm so busy . . . ," "Well, I'm absolutely exhausted . . . ," "I'm up to my neck in it here."

Sound familiar? It's tempting to play the "my time is so precious" game. We kid ourselves that telling everyone how busy we are defines us as important. But being overwhelmed is not a badge of honor—if you are the most drained, overworked person on the planet, does it make you the winner? No. Engaging in destructive one-upmanship scores you neither sympathy nor kudos: it merely creates tension that drains your energy even more.

It's more impressive to be the most relaxed person in the room, to be the person who's got themselves together, who can walk out of the office with a cheery goodbye. That person could be you.

Stop stress taking hold
Adopt power posture and you'll sit less stressed

✓ Sit straight with the top of your monitor at eye level.

✓ Tuck your feet under your desk and place them flat on the floor. Try to catch yourself every time you cross your legs.

✓ You should be able to type without moving your elbows away from your torso.

✗ If your shoulders are hunched, your chin is jutting out or you're bending your head downwards, run through this checklist again.

Hunching down to look at your phone puts up to 60lb of pressure on your spine—ouch! [3].

Keep your head high, squeeze your shoulder blades together and raise your smartphone to meet your gaze, and you won't have to sacrifice your Instagram habit.

Try the 60-second headache soother

Medication isn't the most effective way to treat tension headaches [3]. This stretch is, and it's discreet enough to do sitting at your desk.

● Pull your shoulders back. With your left hand, hold the base of your chair.

● Place your right hand on top of your head and gently press above your left ear, like in this picture. A stretch should be felt on the left side of your neck. Hold for three long, deep breaths.

● Now tuck your chin in and look towards your right hip pocket. You'll feel the stretch all the way down to your left shoulder.

● Hold for another three breaths, then switch sides.

When work is crazy, 15-minute blasts will keep your fitness up. This boosts productivity enough to make up for time out of the office, too [4]

Avoid tucking your phone between your head and shoulder. If you need both hands free while you're on a call, get a headset.

EAT UP YOUR TO-DO LIST

We eat up to three times more at work than we do at home [5].
Tell temptation who's boss with this productivity menu

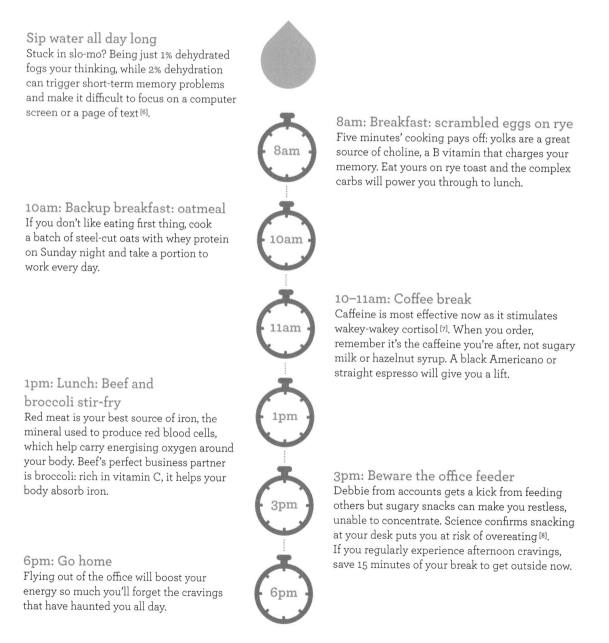

Sip water all day long
Stuck in slo-mo? Being just 1% dehydrated fogs your thinking, while 2% dehydration can trigger short-term memory problems and make it difficult to focus on a computer screen or a page of text [6].

8am: Breakfast: scrambled eggs on rye
Five minutes' cooking pays off: yolks are a great source of choline, a B vitamin that charges your memory. Eat yours on rye toast and the complex carbs will power you through to lunch.

10am: Backup breakfast: oatmeal
If you don't like eating first thing, cook a batch of steel-cut oats with whey protein on Sunday night and take a portion to work every day.

10–11am: Coffee break
Caffeine is most effective now as it stimulates wakey-wakey cortisol [7]. When you order, remember it's the caffeine you're after, not sugary milk or hazelnut syrup. A black Americano or straight espresso will give you a lift.

1pm: Lunch: Beef and broccoli stir-fry
Red meat is your best source of iron, the mineral used to produce red blood cells, which help carry energising oxygen around your body. Beef's perfect business partner is broccoli: rich in vitamin C, it helps your body absorb iron.

3pm: Beware the office feeder
Debbie from accounts gets a kick from feeding others but sugary snacks can make you restless, unable to concentrate. Science confirms snacking at your desk puts you at risk of overeating [8]. If you regularly experience afternoon cravings, save 15 minutes of your break to get outside now.

6pm: Go home
Flying out of the office will boost your energy so much you'll forget the cravings that have haunted you all day.

You wear a good night's sleep like a superhero cape
– it makes you feel like you can take on the world.

And when you don't have a good night, it sets a gloomy tone for your whole day. We overreact to small problems and take less notice of good things going on. We skip our workout, then eat all the wrong things and feel worse [1].

"Well, I'm just a bad sleeper," you say, matchsticks weighed down by the weight of your eyelids. But you don't have to muddle through: let's find out what's going on with your body now. Keep a notebook next to your bed.

Every night, jot down …
1. What did you eat this evening and when?

2. What were you doing tonight before bed?

3. How do you feel, in one word?

In the morning note three things:
1. When did you get into bed and when did you turn the lights off?

2. What time did you wake up?

3. What word describes your mood this morning?

If you're tired right now, the mere idea of keeping a sleep diary may sound ridiculous. But it's your best hope of sorting out your slumber so give it a try, just for a week [2]

After a week (probably sooner), you'll spot patterns that help you to see how your food, stress levels and timings impact your sleep.

In this chapter, you'll find practical advice that helps you eat to support good sleep, de-compress before bed and—while you're still struggling to switch off—learn how to survive a sleep-deprived day.

Four simple words that will help you consistently get the right amount of sleep: get to bed earlier

- Keeping a regular sleep schedule helps your body clock switch on and off at the right time, which means you're less likely to be awake when you don't want to be.

- Use 1% of your day to help: aim to get into bed 15 minutes earlier each day until you're in bed, lights out, at 10pm.

- Should you need another incentive, it's nice to know that people who go to bed and wake up at about the same time each day have lower body fat than those with more erratic schedules [3].

Trust these tried-and-tested accessories to help you produce more melatonin, the sleepy hormone:

Blackout blinds or a sleep mask. Make your bedroom as pitch black as possible—your body only produces melatonin in the dark. If your optic nerve detects light, you will wake up [4].
Loose PJs. Tight clothing can curb melatonin production by 60% [5].

And avoid these:
Your phone, laptop, tablet or TV. Switch them off and you'll switch off too. Electronic devices emit a short-wavelength light, even on standby mode, that interferes with melatonin production [6].

Tired? Invest 15 minutes of your evening and go to bed earlier

THE SECRET LIFE OF YOUR SLEEPING BODY

While you're dreaming about zombies, your body is ticking through its to-do list. Use this timeline to take advantage of the best time to go to bed and wake up

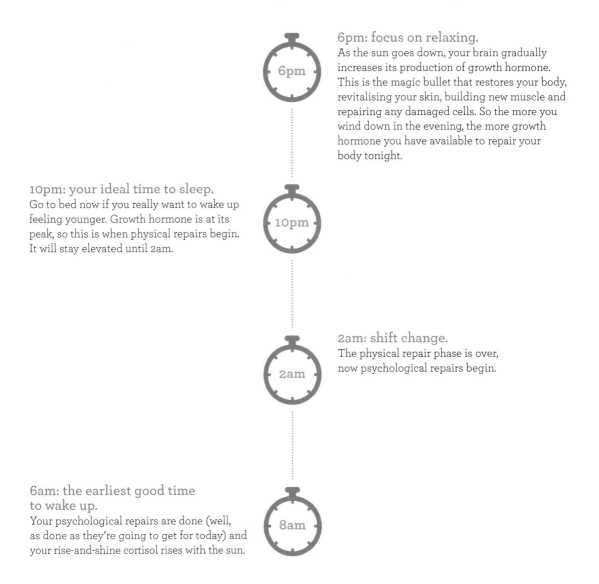

6pm: focus on relaxing.
As the sun goes down, your brain gradually increases its production of growth hormone. This is the magic bullet that restores your body, revitalising your skin, building new muscle and repairing any damaged cells. So the more you wind down in the evening, the more growth hormone you have available to repair your body tonight.

10pm: your ideal time to sleep.
Go to bed now if you really want to wake up feeling younger. Growth hormone is at its peak, so this is when physical repairs begin. It will stay elevated until 2am.

2am: shift change.
The physical repair phase is over, now psychological repairs begin.

6am: the earliest good time to wake up.
Your psychological repairs are done (well, as done as they're going to get for today) and your rise-and-shine cortisol rises with the sun.

The 3-minute sleep trick that makes you wake refreshed

Do these three stretches in bed to bring oxygen to tired muscles and calm cortisol, so your racing mind can relax

Hug it out

Lie on your back in bed and take a deep breath, filling your belly with air. As you slowly exhale, hug your right knee into your chest. Think of it as a bellow, pushing stale air out of your body. Inhale, releasing your right knee. Repeat another nine times. Keep your left leg flat on the floor until you've hugged your right knee ten times, then switch.

Twist away tension

Still lying on your back, bend your knees so both feet are flat on the floor. Stretch your arms wide, palms up. Inhale deeply, then let your knees fall to the right so they're bent at 90° and stacked on top of each other. Gently turn your head to gaze at your left hand and take four more deep diaphragmatic breaths. Progress the stretch by straightening your top leg, and slowly take another five deep breaths. Switch sides and repeat.

Beditate

This deep diaphragmatic breath is also known as ocean breathing or *ujjayi* in yoga. Inhale through the nose, filling your lower belly, lower rib cage, then up to your chest and throat. Exhale through the nose for a count of three. Keep a steady rhythm as you repeat the movement. Counting to ten—one as you inhale, two as you exhale—might help you focus. If you lose count, or when you get to ten, simply start again. Sleep is within touching distance.

In one groundbreaking study, soldiers with post-traumatic stress practised this breath exercise for up to an hour a day. After a month, 90% of them felt well [7]. If simply breathing can do that for them— some of the most stressed-out people on the planet who have borne witness to utter horror—what could it do for you?

Bug-eyed at 3am? Read this

It's normal to wake in the night, but our conscious minds start to worry about sleeping. Ironically, that's what keeps us awake. The stress of sleeplessness becomes a self-fulfilling prophecy: spikes in cortisol make you wired and unable to sleep. The secret to getting a good night's shut-eye is to set yourself up for relaxation, then do nothing—just lie back and let it happen.

DO: Remember good rest beats poor sleep
Tell yourself it doesn't matter if you don't sleep tonight, you'll just use the time to rest. You'll be surprised how quickly you get to sleep when you take the pressure off.

DO: Boycott the bedroom
Tossing and turning for hours stresses you out and actually keeps you awake. Pottering around another room for 20 minutes—a technique called sleep restriction—will speed your return to slumber [8]. When you get back into bed, you're relaxed and less afraid of sleeplessness.

DON'T: Start the day any time before 6am
So hands off your phone, as it overstimulates your brain, and don't turn on the TV as it will put your mind in daytime mode. The best restful distractions are reading a book or listening to music.

Saying thank you can help even the hardiest insomniac

When you get into bed, think of five good things that happened today. Perhaps you got a text that made you smile or finished a piece of work you're proud of. Remember all the 1% blocks you've invested in making yourself feel better today. Listing reasons to be thankful drops your stress levels almost immediately, even if you're a die-hard cynic, rolling your eyes as you read this. Commit to trying this for 21 days and you'll notice the difference.

YOUR GOOD SLEEP MENU

If you're too full, you'll toss and turn for hours. If you haven't eaten enough, you'll wake up hungry. Here's what to eat…

IF DINNER WAS TOO LONG AGO

You can't drop off on an empty tummy, so have a sleepy snack:

- **Avocado and turkey on crackers—** the perfect combination of tryptophan, protein, healthy fats and just a little carbs.
- **Cashew oatmeal—**oats aren't just for breakfast. They contain melatonin and complex carbs that can help more tryptophan flow into your brain. Meanwhile, the warm milk helps you sleep (it's not just an old wives' tale) and a sprinkle of cashews on top supply zinc. Deficiency of this mineral is linked to night wakings.

IF YOU HAVE TO HAVE A LATE DINNER

We know eating late isn't ideal, but sometimes we have no choice. The secret is to eat easy-to-digest foods. Take your pick:

- **Kale omelette with cheese—**cheese won't give you nightmares and this dish is rich in calcium and the amino acid tryptophan, which your brain needs to manufacture the sleepy hormone melatonin. Cue a snoozy, satisfied sensation.
- **Salmon miso soup with spinach—** salmon is high in vitamin B6, a building block of the sleepy hormone melatonin. Poach it in miso, which is high in tryptophan, then garnish with calcium-pumped spinach.

[...] ND SOLUTIONS

- **S[...]** you up when your b[...] Brew a cup of camomile, as thi[...]s off your urge to OD on sugar. [...]reams.
- **Red meat and raw veg[...]s—**foods that sit too heavily in you[...]ach or take too long to digest will kee[...]p. Drink peppermint tea, it's like a n[...]ntacid that relaxes your digestive sy[...]

Sleep off your spare tire

A sleep deficit makes your body produce more cortisol, the stress hormone that triggers storage of excess fat around your stomach. Getting an extra 90 minutes' sleep a night not only makes you feel 14% less hungry, but also means you eat more nutritious food—one study shows a 62% fall in cravings for junk food [9].

Never use a sleep tracker

In order to sleep, you need to stop measuring and let go. Trackers turn sleep into a high-pressure event. It's normal to wake up during the night, but if you look at data in that time, your brain switches on and will take ages to get back to deep delta sleep.

Like energy, willpower fades during the day

So it pays to be more aware that when you're tired, your feelgood guard is down and cravings may intensify. We often misinterpret this search for evening energy as an excuse to fill our bellies with sugary Crunchy Nut Cornflakes. In fact, your body is simply saying "go to bed".

If evening is the only time you can exercise …

Do a less intense workout than you would normally, and calm your cortisol straight afterwards with extra stretches, a hot meal, candlelight, an Epsom salt bath and your favorite chill-out tunes. Throw everything at it. If you can only ever exercise in the evening and it's compromising your sleep, shift your workout schedule around so you do more at the weekend and less Monday to Friday.

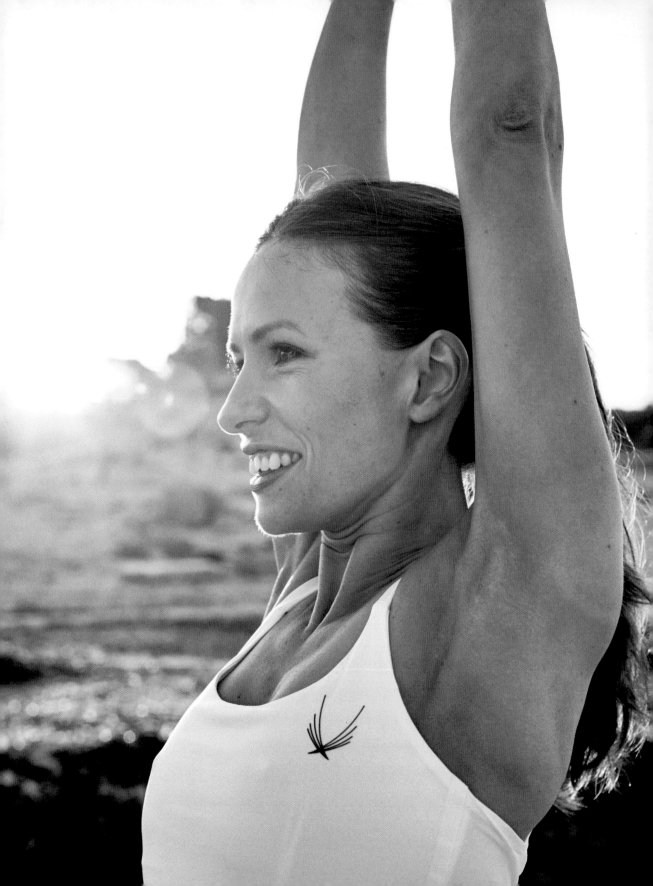

PART 5

12-WEEK PLAN

If you're tired of feeling tired, if you're unhappy with your body and your moods are all over the place, this plan will help you get back to happy

BYE, RUT. THIS PLAN WILL LIFT YOU UP, UP, UP

The 12-week feelgood plan eases you in v-e-r-y gently, and every step is doable.
In the next 84 days, you'll set up the structure that makes being healthy feel effortless.
And you'll begin to feel better from the moment you start making healthy changes.

Here's how you can expect your life to improve:
* You'll develop an easy-going, happy relationship with food.
* You're likely to drop two dress sizes if you have the excess weight to lose,
  and you'll certainly get "you-look-great" fitter.
* You'll sleep better, have more energy and generally be in a better mood.

START HERE Set your goal
I want

and I *know* it will make me feel good

Gather your kit:
☑ Download an interval timer on your smartphone
☑ Pack your gym bag
☑ Have your diary poised to enter workouts into your calendar

Take a selfie—12 weeks from now you're going to be pretty happy with this
because you'll see how far you've come. Note down your measurements too

Weight:

Waist:

Thighs:

Upper arms:

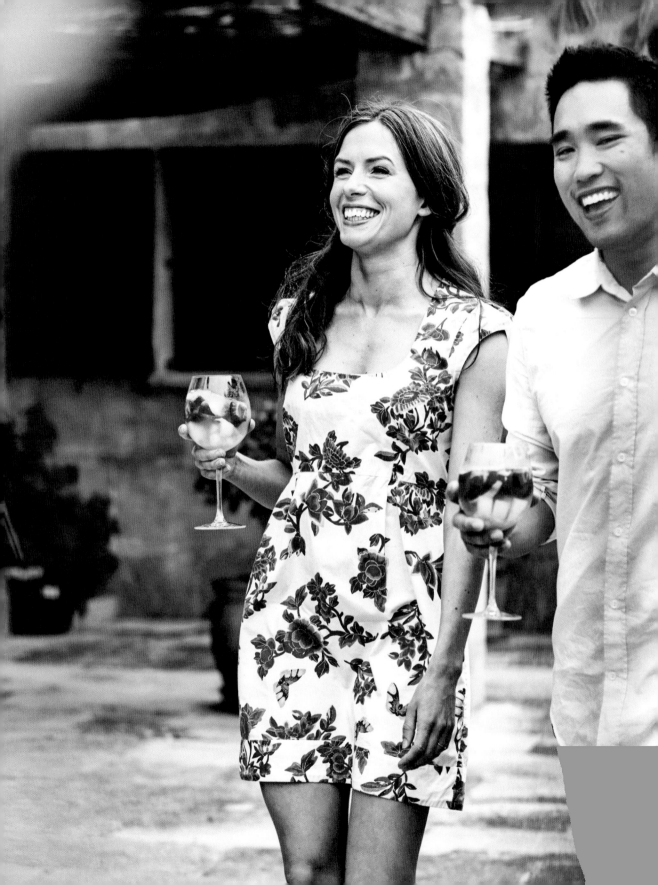

WEEK 1

Your first step is to ID exactly what's getting in the way of you feeling good

BECOME A FOOD FORENSIC

* Note down everything you eat and drink, just for a week. This is your chance to look at the food you like to eat every day and identify tweaks to make it healthier. A much happier alternative to trying to live on a restrictive diet! Keep your journal simple—try this:

When did you eat?

What did you eat?

Did you enjoy your food?

How did you feel at the time?

How did you feel afterwards?

* If you're already thinking this looks like too much, take photos and make notes on your smartphone. This is your diary—keep it however works best for you.

* The idea is to understand the link between food and your emotions, so you start to feed your body the nourishing food it needs. Being tuned in means you'll also break down the habit of eating when you're not hungry.

* This diary is supposed to be a picture of what's going on in your life right now, but if you instinctively find yourself being more mindful, that's totally fine: you're improving already.

Keeping a diary sounds like a hassle...

Come on. It takes less than a minute to jot down what you're eating, and mere seconds to note the time you turn the lights off at night. In the time it took you to decide you didn't have time to write down what you ate, you could have done it already.

Remember: you're doing this for yourself. This diary is important. It will give you the tangible grasp on reality you need to become mindful of what's really happening with your body.

SCHEDULE SHORT WORKOUTS

* Start with the Anti-Ager workout plan—turn to page 131 for all the details.

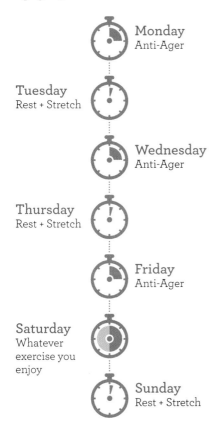

Monday
Anti-Ager

Tuesday
Rest + Stretch

Wednesday
Anti-Ager

Thursday
Rest + Stretch

Friday
Anti-Ager

Saturday
Whatever exercise you enjoy

Sunday
Rest + Stretch

* If you're pretty fit already and the first Anti-Ager workout is a breeze, accelerate your progress with another 15 minutes, incorporating the weights and progressions on page 139. If you still feel good on Sunday, next week you can go straight to the Espresso Energizer (see page 141).

KEEP A SLEEP DIARY AND HAVE A MASSAGE

* Observing the pattern between your mood, timings and stress levels for a week will lay the foundation for consistently getting better sleep. Your diary takes less than a minute—here's what to do:

Every night, jot down ...
1. What did you eat this evening and when?

2. What were you doing tonight before bed?

3. How do you feel, in one word?

In the morning note three things:
1. When did you get into bed and when did you turn the lights off?

2. What time did you wake up?

3. What word describes your mood this morning?

* To celebrate your first week on the plan, treat yourself to a massage. Any calming treatment is good, but the best is a lymphatic drainage massage as it stimulates a natural detox, which helps reset your body.

Wake up your breakfast, step away from your cravings and set the scene for a good night's sleep

EAT

PLAY BREAKFAST ROULETTE

* Start bettering your diet with breakfast, because a good morning meal is the key to eating well all day. This week you'll try seven different healthy breakfasts to see how your body responds (see below).

* Tick the breakfasts you like on this chart. When you struggle in the next few weeks, come back to them.

	DID YOU ENJOY YOUR FOOD?	DOES IT SATISFY YOU AND GIVE YOU ENERGY?	CAN YOU LAST UNTIL LUNCH WITHOUT A SNACK?
Monday—Greek yogurt with blueberries, raspberries and chia seeds and a green juice	○	○	○
Tuesday—Rye toast with cashew butter and a green juice	○	○	○
Wednesday—Home-made oatmeal with pumpkin seeds and almonds and a green juice	○	○	○
Thursday—Smoked salmon, sliced avocado and spinach on wheat toast	○	○	○
Friday—Berry smoothie bowl with raspberries, almonds and coconut with a green juice	○	○	○
Saturday—Poached eggs on buttered rye with watercress and hand-carved ham	○	○	○
Sunday—Protein pancakes with strawberries and blackberries and a green juice	○	○	○

* Your how-tos—as well as many more options—are in the breakfast feelgood grid on page 44. What you want to include is: protein, complex carbs, healthy fat and green leafy vegetables. It doesn't matter whether you eat your vegetables or drink them—either is fine.

* Look back at last week's food diary, paying particular attention to what you ate, how much and how you felt afterwards. Put question marks next to things you're not sure are great for you. This activity sets mindfulness into motion.

WORK OUT IN FRONT OF THE MIRROR AND WALK OFF CRAVINGS

* This week, do your Anti-Aging circuits in a mirror so you can focus on getting great form. Note how your muscles engage and your posture opens up when you do moves as they're meant to be done. This is the key to toning up: you target the muscles you want to use and avoid injury. Once you've nailed form, you can increase the intensity of your workout—do more reps in each minute, add a weight, or both. These progressions will get you   more results.

* Does the Anti-Ager circuit feel too easy? Use the upgrades on page 139 to get ready for the Espresso Energizer.

* Be careful not to overcompensate for the effort you put into exercise by snacking. Ask yourself if you're truly hungry, or maybe just thirsty—the two are easily confused. When a snack attack strikes, take a walk. Striding for 15 minutes can see off cravings. If you're ravenous after your stroll, nibble on air-popped popcorn or a palmful of pumpkin seeds and blueberries. Flick to the top ten snacks with feelgood superpowers on page 88.

SET YOUR SLEEP SCENE

* Analyse last week's sleep diary. Is there a correlation between how late you turn the lights off and how rested you feel in the morning? Is there a link between doing work in the evening and having a restless night? This week you're going to experiment with a wind-down pattern that will help you be more mindful of those connections and improve the quality of your sleep.

* Kit yourself out with a sleep mask, blackout blinds or both. The darker you make your bedroom, the sounder your sleep could be. A few drops of soothing lavender or orange blossom oil on your pillow can help, too.

* Regenerate with an Epsom salts bath once or twice a week. A cup of these magnesium-rich salts in your bathwater helps soak soreness from your muscles, drains a bloated tummy, smoothes cellulite and helps you sleep, too.

No time to train?

It's only 15 minutes, three times a week! That's 1% of your day dedicated to making you feel good. You can do it in your underwear. You can do it in the privacy of your own home. You can do it in front of the TV. You can do it as slowly as your body needs today. Ultimately, you can do it!

You already feel better and sleep better and you're only a quarter of the way through. Get ready to up your game

EAT

PLAY THE LUNCH LOTTERY

* Now you know what breakfasts work, eat them. Add your new ingredients to your regular shopping list.

* Try seven different feelgood lunches to see what fits with your routine, palate and body. Keep true to your normal habits, so let's assume you want to grab something convenient Monday to Friday, and you're happy cooking at the weekend.

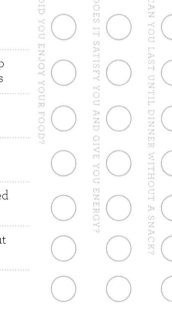

Monday—Supermarket salad bowl with an extra chicken breast. Use half the dressing and spritz fresh lemon instead

Tuesday—Rainbow vegetable meze of yellow pepper, sugar snap peas, carrots, beetroot, black olives and cucumber, with hummus

Wednesday—Salad Niçoise. Add extra tinned tuna if the salad you buy isn't big enough

Thursday—Mushroom, red pepper and cheese omelette with a big green salad

Friday—Sashimi with a big miso soup, seaweed salad and pickled ginger

Saturday—Tom yum soup with prawns, bok choy and mangetout

Sunday—Roast chicken with steamed Savoy cabbage, peas, purple sprouting broccoli and roast sweet potato

Column headers: DID YOU ENJOY YOUR FOOD? / DOES IT SATISFY YOU AND GIVE YOU ENERGY? / CAN YOU LAST UNTIL DINNER WITHOUT A SNACK?

* You've got more lunch options in the feelgood grid on page 52. The basic formula is to eat plenty of vegetables and protein, add a little complex carbs like sweet potato and enjoy a little healthy fat like olive oil dressing. If you crave a sweet taste afterwards, brew a cup of tea.

* Tick the lunches that work for you. Remember these meals when you're stuck for a healthy lunch in the future.

SWEAT MINDFULLY AND SWITCH CLASSES

* By now you'll start seeing results from the exercise you're doing, so it's the perfect time to enhance your mindfulness. Observe that your workouts feel easier, even the exercises you found difficult at first. Your muscles feel stronger. Notice how you drop deeper into a stretch and lower into a squat. Observe that your clothes fit better. Pay attention to the difference it makes to your lunge when you engage your core. Thrill in the moment you feel endorphins start to flow, and you'll feel good.

* Hopefully you'll feel ready to advance to the Espresso Energizer workout next week, so use the upgrades on page 147 to build some upward momentum. But if your muscles are in any pain, it's totally OK to stay at the Anti-Ager plan for another week.

* The freestyle workout is a key part of your fitness plan: it's all about releasing feelgood endorphins that make you love exercise a little bit more. If you're half-hearted about going to a gym class you thought you'd enjoy, switch. Try a new class (you don't have to do your freestyle workout on Saturday), get active with a friend or use that hour to explore a new part of your neighbourhood on a run.

THE 15-MINUTE SECRET TO GETTING MORE SLEEP

* Now you've found your ultimate unwind routine, bring your bedtime forward by 15 minutes each night until you're in bed by 10pm. Set an alarm to remind yourself to wind down, if you find it hard to remember. By the end of the week you'll go to bed when you're tired in the evening, instead of pushing through for a second wind and feeling horrible the next day.

* If your social life gets in the way one or two nights of the week, don't worry. Just set your evening alarm 15 minutes earlier so you reset the following evening. If you're out late every night, take a moment to rethink why feeling good is important to you—go back to your pledge at the beginning of this plan to get your head straight.

What if you can't find a healthy lunch anywhere?

Then you make your own and bring it to work in a lunchbox. Are you OK feeling lousy every afternoon because of the greasy lunch options at the deli? If not, then make a positive change.

WEEK 4

You've got this far, so you can get to week 12. You're already feeling better: you've got more energy, more patience, a better sex drive. Here's how to keep up the feelgood buzz

EAT

FIND WINNING DINNERS

* Now you've got four or five great go-tos for effortlessly easy feelgood breakfasts and lunches. Eat up!

* This week, observe what a nourishing evening meal does for you. Look at the feelgood dinner grid on page 60 and pick seven different options to throw together this week. Or you could try:

	DID YOU ENJOY YOUR FOOD?	DOES IT SATISFY YOU AND GIVE YOU ENERGY?	CAN YOU LAST UNTIL BEDTIME WITHOUT A SNACK?
Monday—Lemon-baked cod on a pea purée with sweet potato fries and roast rainbow veggies	○	○	○
Tuesday—Organic lamb burger with sweet potato wedges and a big green salad	○	○	○
Wednesday—Cauli risotto primavera with spring onion, spinach, broad beans, collard greens and lemon zest	○	○	○
Thursday—Triple-vitamin chili with ground beef, black beans, leeks, mushrooms, carrots and red peppers on cauli rice	○	○	○
Friday—Mussels in lemony tomato broth with pea shoots, radishes, fennel, leeks and rye bread	○	○	○
Saturday—Chicken tikka with red lentil dahl and raw Indian salad	○	○	○
Sunday—Lamb tagine with butternut squash, onion, tomato, green pepper, eggplant and quinoa	○	○	○

* The basic rule is this: more protein, plenty of vegetables, some healthy fats like avocado, salmon, olive oil or coconut oil.

* Tick the meals that make you feel good so you remember them in future.

* To see how your menu fits around social engagements and family commitments, refer back to the feelgood guide to eating out on page 104.

GET A FITNESS PROMOTION AND EAT MORE

* If you aced the Anti-Ager upgrades last week, you're ready for the Espresso Energizer workout plan. Here's your schedule:

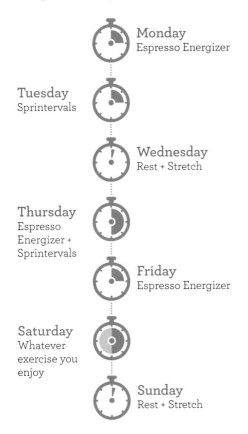

Monday
Espresso Energizer

Tuesday
Sprintervals

Wednesday
Rest + Stretch

Thursday
Espresso Energizer + Sprintervals

Friday
Espresso Energizer

Saturday
Whatever exercise you enjoy

Sunday
Rest + Stretch

* Yes, it's as little as 1 hour 45 minutes a week. Turn to page 141 for the nitty-gritty.

STRETCH YOURSELF TO SLEEP

* If it takes you a while to sleep, deepen your wind-down with a soporific series of knee hugs, tension-easing twists and beditation breaths. It takes 3 minutes and the technique is on page 182.

* On evenings when you have more time, treat yourself to a hot bath with Epsom salts. Soaking in these magnesium salts once or twice every week not only helps you sleep, but also boosts blood flow to knotted muscles.

You might get hungrier now.

That's totally cool: you're burning more calories, so you need more. Just be sure to feed your hunger with nourishing food. So no, fries don't count. And while you get used to the workouts, treat yourself to more sleep.

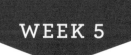

Crack your snack habit, stay on the fit track and discover what's really stressing you out

EAT

SORT OUT SNACKS AND DRINK WATER IN DISGUISE

* Your personal feelgood menu is set up and you're eating three good meals a day. But if your healthy meals are being undermined by a less-than-healthy snacking habit, focus on hydration. Thirst is often mistaken for hunger, so make water your first go-to when a snack attack hits. H2O makes every single cell in your body function better, so being well-hydrated helps you feel energized, calm and in control. Sip water in several different forms—sparkling, herbal tea, fruit-infused—before you reach for a snack, and you may find you don't need that sticky cereal bar so badly
after all.

* If you are genuinely hungry, it may be because your last meal wasn't good enough, so stay mindful of how satisfied you are after eating. Unsurprisingly, hunger is also a side-effect of leaving too long between meals. If this is the way your schedule works, fine. Just be sure to feed your body with nourishing snacks like Greek yogurt, air-popped popcorn or apple slices with cashew butter—see page 88 for more smart snacking options.

Snack SOS

If you're a lifelong snacker, it's going to take a while to train your brain out of the habit. Break each craving down one by one, and your new healthy habits will take root.

THREE WAYS TO FIT FITNESS INTO YOUR LIFE

* If exercise is taking up too much of your time, prioritize high-intensity training for faster impact. Now you're fitter, cut down your rest time by 10 seconds between sprints and keep cutting until you feel challenged.

* If now never feels like the perfect time to exercise, remember that a workout always feels better on the other side. In the time it takes to procrastinate, you could have finished training already. The solution? Start your warm-up, however you feel, and the rest will follow. Even 1 minute is better than nothing at all. No one ever regrets a workout: you always feel better for doing it.

* If you're struggling to train because you feel sore, don't worry. It's a sign your muscles are activating. And you went up a level last week, so you are challenging yourself. Add another round of warm-up stretches before every workout to boost healing blood flow where it's needed.

ACTIVELY DE-STRESS

* Your body absorbs stress like a sponge, often making a tricky situation even harder to deal with, and giving you a "tension hangover" long after the crisis has passed. Stop stress becoming a pain in your neck by foam rolling stiff shoulders and sore backs. All you need is a wall, a tennis ball and the guide on page 170.

* If you suffer bloating and stomach cramps when you're stressed, you can tackle them hands-on, too. Your how-to is on page 169.

Accelerate your goals with these fine-tuning tricks

EAT

UPGRADE YOUR BREAKFAST

* You've had 4 weeks of eating good breakfasts, but two small tweaks will make you feel even better.

* Firstly, try swapping out some of your carbs and eating more protein. For example, substitute a slice of rye bread for an extra scrambled egg, or halve the amount of oats in your oatmeal and add an extra sprinkle of nuts, chia or pumpkin seeds.

* Secondly, add some more leafy greens to power up your morning with extra nutrients. Throw a handful of arugula onto your omelette, whiz up a green juice with watercress and celery, or pop a cube of frozen spinach into your pancake batter.

MOVE

GENERATE EXTRA ENERGY

* Switch your workout up a gear so you're ready to start Power Circuits next week. Use the progressions on page 147 to supercharge every move in your Espresso Energizer circuit.

RELAX

CLEAR YOUR HEAD BEFORE BED

* Wipe worries away from your day by focusing on what you have to be grateful for. When you get into bed, think of five good things that happened today. Perhaps a colleague made you a cup of tea unprompted, you saw a silly video that made you laugh, or you ate strawberries that tasted of pure sunshine. Mentally noting reasons to be thankful drops your stress levels almost immediately, even if you're thinking "what the *what*?" as you read this. Where positive thoughts flow, good sleep follows.

Don't forget to stretch on your rest days

Stretching elongates your muscles and encourages restorative blood flow to your tone-me-up hotspots. It's the best way to keep your body working in tip-top condition.

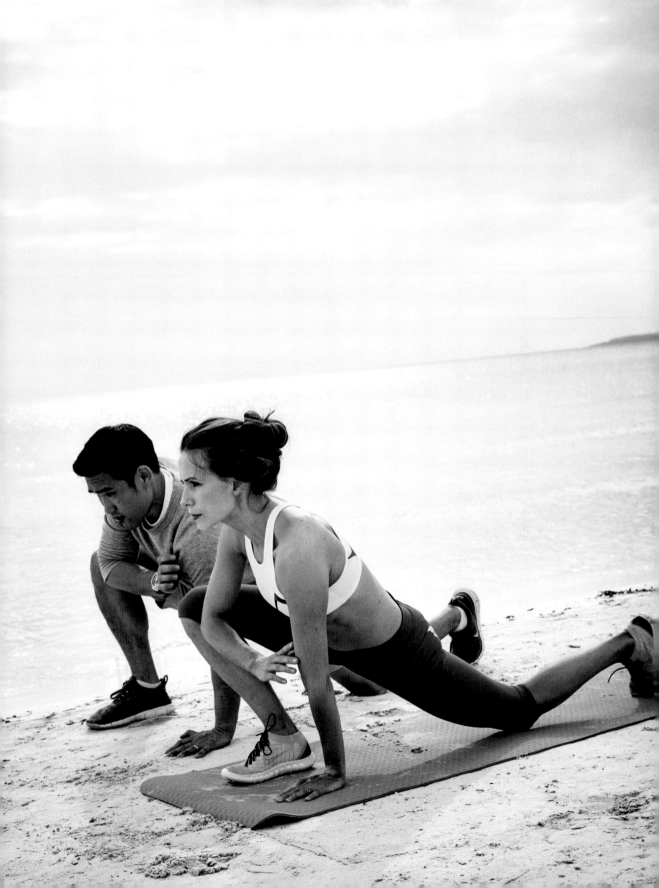

WEEK 7

The secret to enjoying luxurious lunches, powering up your workouts and sleeping soundly

EAT

LIFT LUNCH UP TO THE NEXT LEVEL

✳ Now you're in a rhythm of eating a good lunch, ask yourself how can you make it better. Aim to halve your amount of convenience lunches so you know exactly what ingredients you're eating. Also, buying a nutritious lunch on the go tends to be expensive, which may thwart your healthy intentions by the end of the month. So make your own and pack your lunchbox with ingredients to enhance your day. Turn back to the feelgood grid on page 52 for nutritious DIY lunch ideas. You can throw together a delicious lunch from staple ingredients in your fridge in as little as 2 minutes, so don't worry about eating up your time.

✳ Save even more time by reworking a portion of your dinner for tomorrow's lunch. Freshening up the format breathes new life into your leftovers:

– Pop your ingredients in a corn tortilla and create wraps;

– Serve meat or fish on a bed of salad or roast vegetables;

– Switch the sauce: lemon juice, olive oil and vinegar works with pretty much everything;

– Wrap your ingredients in sheets of nori and dip them in soy sauce, sushi style;

– Add stock to make a simple soup.

MOVE

GET POWERFUL

* If you're comfortable with the Espresso Energizer progressions from last week, your body is ready to get stuck into this power plan. All the details you need are on page 151.

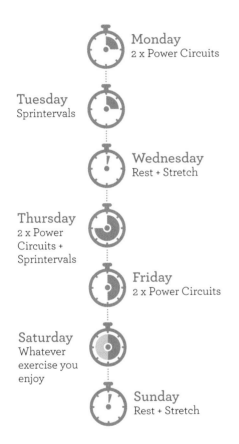

Monday
2 x Power Circuits

Tuesday
Sprintervals

Wednesday
Rest + Stretch

Thursday
2 x Power Circuits + Sprintervals

Friday
2 x Power Circuits

Saturday
Whatever exercise you enjoy

Sunday
Rest + Stretch

RELAX

OBSERVE A CAFFEINE CURFEW

* The beauty of eating better and exercising more is that you'll naturally have more energy. So now's the perfect time to cut down on caffeine—it's one of the most effective ways to improve the quality of your sleep.

* You probably know to avoid coffee after 2pm, but if you're having trouble going to sleep you may be extra-sensitive to the stimulant. Cut out other culprits like chocolate, cola (including diet cola), green tea and painkillers in the evening.

* You can drink a surprising amount of coffee: research shows the average person can drink 400mg—that's two standard barista coffees—to get all the benefits and none of the jittery, stressed-out side-effects [1]. Cut down by a cup a day until you're comfortably within the limit.

Are you ready?

If you're still working on those progressions, wait another week. Mix up your sprintervals, so if you usually run, switch to swimming, cycling or using a rowing machine. A fresh twist in your routine will keep your fitness moving forward.

Batch-cook like a boss, resist seconds, lift more
and regenerate your body

EAT

DOUBLE-DUTY DINNERS

* Big is best when it comes to cooking. Home-made meals are always better than convenience food because you can choose exactly what you want to eat. But cooking can be time-consuming, so if your working week is hectic, set aside an hour at the weekend to batch-cook and stash portions in the freezer. See page 68 for freezer-friendly ideas.

Portion control

If cooking in bulk means eating in bulk, here's what to do:

* Box up your lunchbox and freezer portions now—they're not for picking at.

* When you've finished eating, get up from the table so you don't idly pop another spoonful in your mouth.

* Make yourself a cup of your favorite herbal tea (peppermint and chamomile are best for after dinner) to mark the end of your meal.

* Thinking of an activity you enjoy can fight your urge to grab a rogue forkful, so visualize swinging in a hammock or chatting to your parents.

* If you still can't take the heat, get out of the kitchen for at least 15 minutes. Take a walk, listen to music or prep your gym bag for tomorrow.

MOVE

GO FOR THE GAINS

* If the Power Circuits already feel easy (champ!), increase your weights, cram more reps into each minute, do an extra round of each move, or do all of these things. Small changes get big results. See the progression suggestions on page 159.

RELAX

YES, YOU DESERVE A MASSAGE

* After 8 weeks of training, regeneration is vital. You're already soaking in an Epsom salts bath once or twice a week and smoothing out knotted muscles with a tennis ball, but you've totally earned a luxurious soft-tissue massage, too.

* If you're still feeling sore, up your intake of omega-3s, as these essential fatty acids will help fight inflammation. Sprinkle walnuts on your oatmeal, add flaxseed to your green juice, and eat oily fish like salmon, trout or mackerel three times a week.

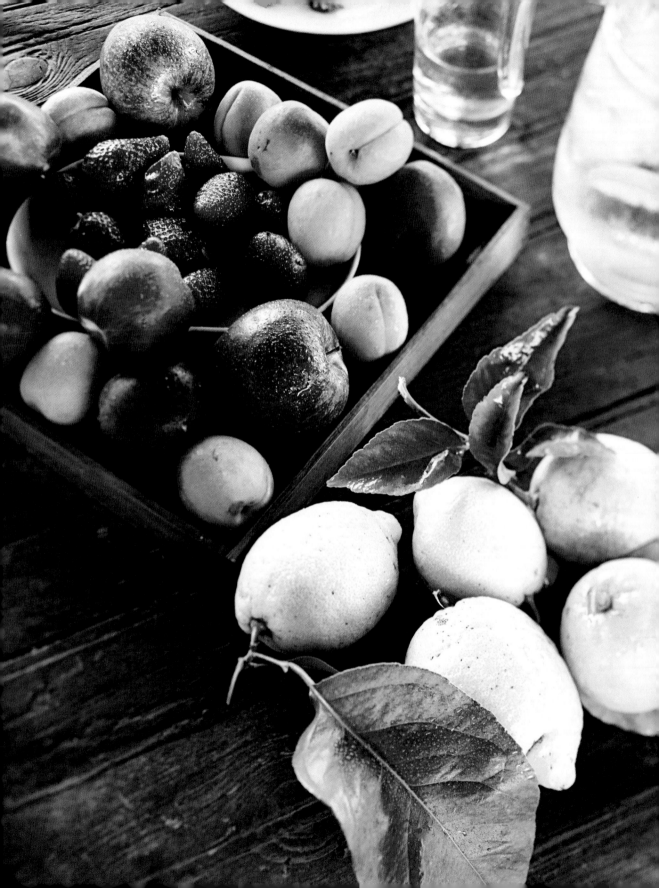

Sort out serving sizes, make more of your rest days
and load up on relax snacks

EAT

PRIORITIZE PORTION CONTROL

* Now you're eating much more nutritious food, it's worth checking your portion sizes. Here's your guide:

Lean meat or oily fish: a deck of cards

Cheese: a matchbox

Sweet potato: a computer mouse

Butter: your thumbnail

Brown rice: a tennis ball

Peanut butter: 2 level tablespoons

Fruit: two cupped handfuls

Olive or coconut oil: 1 tablespoon

Nuts: a palmful

Yogurt: one small cup

Bread: one slice

Oatmeal: ½ cup oats, cooked

Observe that you need less complex carbs on rest days, as your body isn't burning them off. If in doubt, load your plate with extra vegetables.

MOVE

DO ACTIVE RECOVERY ON YOUR REST DAYS

* Take advantage of the fact you've got more energy now and turn your rest time into active recovery days. It's not about pushing yourself—taking a hike with a friend (take a picnic, too, it's not a bootcamp) or going swimming with your family is an endorphin-boosting mental break from your training plan and a chance for your muscles to gently repair themselves.

RELAX

INSTANT ENERGY

* You don't need sugar, you need a calm, clear head. And the best way to get it is with a relax snack: a bite-sized breather. Try the bath breath, energising earlobe trick and more on page 177.

Do nothing

It's tempting to schedule activities for every waking minute in our constantly connected lives, but setting 1% of your day aside—that's just 15 minutes—to be totally idle could be exactly what you need to relax mindfully.

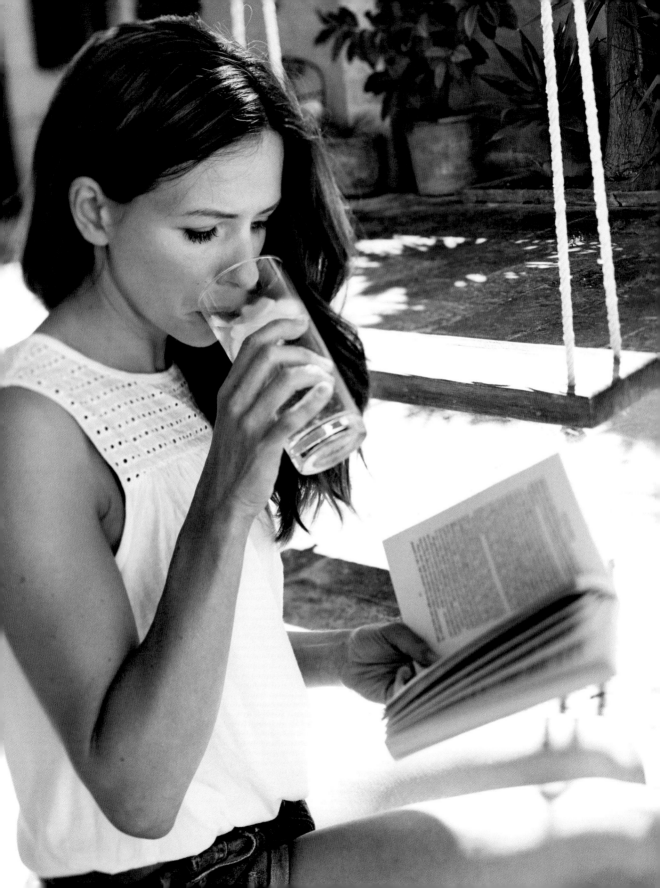

WEEK 10

Snack mindfully, reinvent your cardio and find your power posture

EAT

REVISIT SNACKING

* Healthy snacks can be part of a balanced diet, as long as eating between meals doesn't send you down a slippery slope. This week, every time you crave a snack, use the "Do you really need a snack right now?" guide on page 74 to check if you're definitely hungry, rather than tired, stressed or bored.

Structure your snacks

If you know you need a snack between lunch and dinner, plan what to eat in advance. Having a healthy snack like cashews and blueberries ready will give you the willpower to avoid junk food.

MOVE

DO THE CARDIO --UP

* If you want to put a arugula under your body-sculpting plan, mix up your cardio again. Try skipping, spinning or blasts of butterfly in the pool. Mixing up movement makes your body work in a different way, so you burn more fat.

* If your workout wasn't as good as last time, ask yourself why. Aim for a small improvement with every workout, because that increment is what makes real progress.

RELAX

SIT TALLER

* Your core, back and shoulders are much stronger now, so this week, make a concerted effort to engage those muscles as you sit at your desk with perfect posture. The stresses of your working day will take a far less toll on your body if your back isn't hunched over, your stomach doesn't slump out and your shoulders stay away from your ears. Stick a note to your computer to remind you at regular intervals each day.

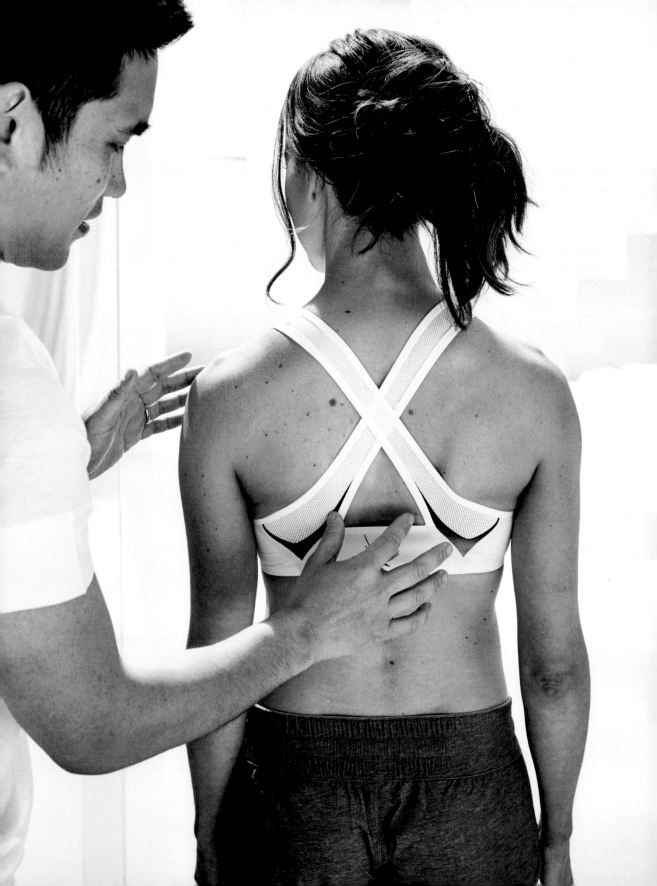

Remember the real world? Get your head back into it.
Also this week: do extra reps and stop feeling tired

EAT

LET GO OF THE GUILT

* You've made lots of healthy, positive changes over the past 9 weeks and you're eating food that makes you feel good. So this is the perfect time to introduce a few not-so-healthy foods—if you like—without undoing the healthy changes you've made. Yes, there is a place for French fries in this plan: it helps keep the feelgood buzz going. In fact, research shows that adding something crave -worthy to your plate can make a healthy meal even more satisfying.

* The key is to enjoy every bite, as it's when we feel guilty for eating the "wrong" thing that we feel out of control and get carried away
by a self-sabotaging urge to overeat. Treat yourself to dinner at your favorite restaurant with friends. Enjoy a few drinks if you like. Take a moment to look around and count your blessings. Indulging occasionally is what makes your healthy habits stick—the odd pizza can make you feel pretty good when the rest of your diet is so wholesome.

MOVE

PUT ON WEIGHTS

* Keep making progress in your circuits by adding more weight to each move: this is what maintains tip-top muscle tone.

* Now you know the moves, use these tricks to work extra reps into your day:

– Squat as you unload the dishwasher;

– Balance in stork stance, eyes closed, as you brush your teeth;

– Bunny-hop up a flight of stairs.

* If lazy habits have crept back in. Don't judge or beat yourself up; simply observe. These observations will create a new template to keep you climbing up the mood curve.

RELAX

STOP FEELING TIRED

* Fatigue is our #1 enemy: it's what makes us produce more cortisol, store excess fat around our middles and chips away at our willpower (did someone say "chips"? Gimme). So if you still feel tired too much of the time, dedicate 1% of your day to freshening up every fatigue flashpoint. Try this:

Within an hour of waking: 15-minute workout—anything from the easy warm-up stretches (page 132) to sprintervals will boost oxygen intake and help see off tiredness.

In the afternoon: brew a green tea, take a head-clearing walk or restore energy by listening to your favorite music.

In the evening: unwind with a 15-minute Epsom salts bath, get into bed quarter of an hour earlier to read—or just turn the light out.

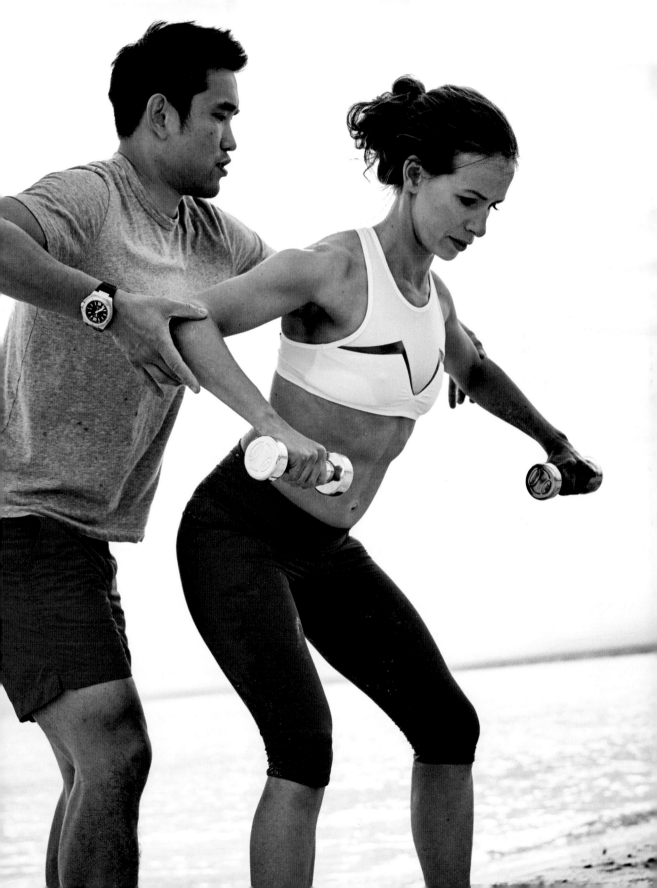

WEEK 12

Whoop! You did it! Right at the top of the feelgood zone, you deserve a gym sabbatical. This week, focus on beating bad habits for good

EAT

MAKE THE FEELGOOD FOOD CONNECTION

* Revisit why you started this plan. Look back at your food diary from week 1 and pat yourself on the back for the positive changes you've made. You've got a better understanding now of what foods make you feel good—sugary cereal for dinner doesn't cut it any more. Maintain that mind/body/energy connection with everything you eat.

MOVE

TAKE A BREAK

* Having 7 days of rest means when you continue your exercise plan next week, you're stronger, which means shooting even higher up the mood curve and constantly getting results. No plateau! Exercise scientists call it "controlled periodisation'. We call it "the easy way to burn more fat and feel even better'.

* If you really love exercise and you feel your stress levels creeping up without your regular workouts, just reduce the intensity by half to give your body a break this week.

RELAX

RESTORE CALM TO YOUR SLEEP ROUTINE

* Go back to your sleep diary from week 1, too—look how tired and cranky you felt back then, and breathe a sigh of relief that fog is lifted.

* If you're still waking up groggy occasionally, plan something worth waking up for every morning, like a detour to the best coffee shop, cooking eggs for breakfast or a new exercise class.

Look at what motivated you to change your life, to have more energy, to feel calmer, to shape up. Are you closer? Add your measurements from week 1 and update your selfie, too. This exercise reinforces how far you've come

WEEK 1

Weight:

Waist:

Thighs:

Upper arms:

WEEK 12

Weight:

Waist:

Thighs:

Upper arms:

Now reset your goal. Having got this far, you realize you can do anything you set your mind to. Aim high!

I want:

…and I know it will make me feel good.

HOW TO FEEL GOOD ALL THE TIME
Keeping up the healthy changes you've made over the last 12 weeks

Over the last 84 days, you've laid down the blueprint for your own personal feelgood plan, and the good news is that it is constantly evolving. You've set up routines and healthy habits that take the stress out of trying to be healthy—in fact, good choices are easy now. You're more aware of what your body is trying to tell you, so when you cut loose, you know how to bounce back into the feelgood zone.

If you're happy with your plan, keep going. If you'd like to go further, do a new food diary this week to look for healthy tweaks, and increase the intensity of your exercise. Lift more weight, add more movement, and keep the combination of strength training and cardio intervals.

The Feelgood Plan is for life
Most diets don't work long-term because as your body changes, your nutritional demands alter, too. When you're fitter, your metabolism is faster and you need to eat more to feed those muscles.

That revelation may feel like a champagne cork popping in your head—or it might make you a little nervous, especially if previous diets have made your weight yo-yo. But the truth is, all the exercise in the world won't work if you're underfed. You can't starve yourself and exercise more: that is a sure-fire route to feeling bad.

So keep checking in on your body. You know how good you feel after a workout, after a good night's sleep, and when you eat healthy, nourishing, real food. You know how bloated, jittery, uncomfortable and tired you feel when you don't exercise, don't sleep, or try to feed your body with processed, sugary, empty energy. But now you have the tools to make the right choice. Do what makes you feel good.

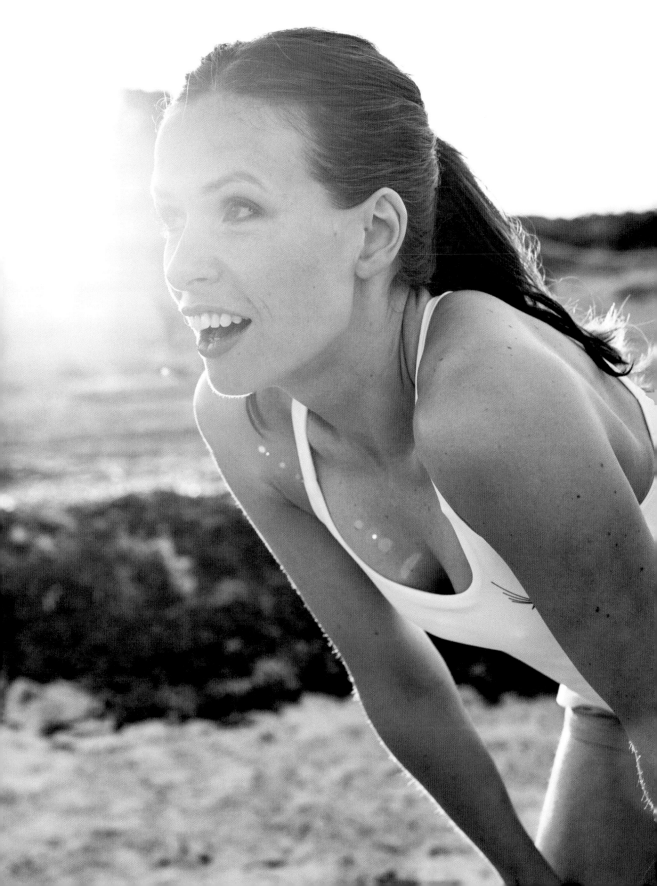

SOURCES

CHAPTER 1

[1] Schmeichel, Brandon J.; Vohs, Kathleen; 2009; "Self-affirmation and self-control: Affirming core values counteracts ego depletion", *Journal of Personality and Social Psychology*, Vol 96(4), Apr 2009, 770–782.

[2] Kuijer RG, Boyce JA; 2014; "Chocolate cake. Guilt or celebration? Associations with healthy eating attitudes, perceived behavioural control, intentions and weight-loss", *Appetite*, 2014 Mar; 74: 48–54

[3] Oswald, A.J,; Proto, E.; Sgroi, D. "Happiness and Productivity' Journal of Labor Economics, 2014

[4] http://www.nhs.uk/conditions/stress-anxiety-depression/pages/feel-better-and-happy.aspx

[5] Puetz TW, Flowers SS, O'Connor PJ. 2008; *Psychotherapy and Psychosomatics*, 2008;77(3):167–74

CHAPTER 2

[1] Pronin E, Olivola CY, Kennedy KA. 2008; *Personality and Social Psychology Bulletin*, "Doing unto future selves as you would do unto others: psychological distance and decision making'

[2] Ersner-Hershfield, H, Elliott Wimmer, G, Knutson, B. 2009; *Social Cognitive and Affective Neuroscience*, "Saving for the future self: Neural measures of future self-continuity predict temporal discounting'; 2009 Mar; 4(1)

[3] Knab AM, Shanely RA, Corbin KD, Jin F, Sha W, Nieman DC; *Medicine & Science in Sports & Exercise*, "A 45-minute vigorous exercise bout increases metabolic rate for 14 hours'; 2011 Sep;43(9):1643-8.

[4] Cosgrove MC1, Franco OH, Granger SP, Murray PG, Mayes AE; *The American Journal of Clinical Nutrition*, "Dietary nutrient intakes and skin-aging appearance among middle-aged American women"; 2007 Oct;86(4): 1225-31.

[5] Möller-Levet CS, Archer SN, Bucca G, Laing EE, Slak A, Kabiljo R, Lo JC, Santhi N, von Schantz M, Smith CP, Dijk DJ.; *Proceedings of the National Academy of Sciences of the United States of America*, "Effects of insufficient sleep on circadian rhythmicity and expression amplitude of the human blood transcriptome" 2013 Mar 19;110(12)

[6] Chollet D, Franken P, Raffin Y, Henrotte JG, Widmer J, Malafosse A, Tafti M; *Behavior Genetics*, "Magnesium involvement in sleep: genetic and nutritional models'; 2001 Sep;31(5):413–25.

[7] Israel, S et al; "Translating Personality Psychology to Help Personalize Preventive Medicine for Young-Adult Patients" *Journal of Personality and Social Psychology*, 2014, Vol. 106(3), 484-498.

CHAPTER 3

[1] Kolotkin R L , Binks M, Crosby R D, Østbye T, Mitchell J E and Hartley G, 2008. "Improvements in sexual quality of life after moderate weight loss, *"International Journal of Impotence Research"*, (2008) 20, 487–492

[2] Research from the National Institute of Clinical Excellence (NICE), 2014.

[3] Dor A, Ferguson C, Langwith C, Tan E, 2010. "A Heavy Burden: The Individual Costs of Being Overweight and Obese in the United States'. *Himmelfarb Health Sciences Library, The George Washington University Health Sciences Research Commons*, September 2010.

[4] Kunikata H1, Watanabe K, Miyoshi M, Tanioka T. 2012. The effects measurement of hand massage by the autonomic activity and psychological indicators. *The Journal of Medical Investigation*, 2012;59(1-2):206-12.

[5] Andrade AM, Greene GW, Melanson KJ. 2008. "Eating slowly led to decreases in energy intake within meals in healthy women'. *Journal of the American Dietetic Association*, 2008 Jul;108(7):1186-91

[6/7] Sherman H, Genzer Y, Cohen R, Chapnik N, Madar Z, Froy O. 2012. "Timed high-fat diet resets circadian metabolism and prevents obesity" *Journal of the Federation of American Societies for Experimental Biology (TheFASEB Journal)* vol. 26 no. 8 3493-3502

CHAPTER 4

[1] Jakubowicz D, Barnea M, Wainstein J, Froy O. 2013. "High caloric intake at breakfast vs. dinner differentially influences weight loss of overweight and obese women", *Obesity*, 2013 Dec;21(12)

[2] Dhurandhar, N, Vander Wal, J S, Currier, N, Khosla, P, Gupta AK. 2007."Egg breakfast enhances weight loss", *The FASEB Journal*, 2007;21:538.1

[3] de la Fuente-Arrillaga, C, et al, 2014. "Glycemic load, glycemic index, bread and incidence of overweight/obesity in a Mediterranean cohort: the SUN project" *BMC Public Health*,2014; 14: 1091.

[4] Malhotra, A, 2013."Saturated fat is not the major issue" *BMJ*, October 2013

[5] Reis, CE, et al. 2013. "Acute and second-meal effects of peanuts on glycaemic response and appetite in obese women with high type 2 diabetes risk: a randomized cross-over clinical trial" *British Journal of Nutrition*, 2013 Jun;109(11), 2015-23.

[6] Rolls, B, 2014. "Cereal flake size influences calorie intake", *Penn State News, 26 March 2014*.

[7] Benbrook, C, et al, 2013. "Organic Production Enhances Milk Nutritional Quality by Shifting Fatty Acid Composition: A United States–Wide, 18-Month Study", *PLOS One*, December 9, 2013

[8] Cameron JD, Cyr MJ, Doucet E. 2010. "Increased meal frequency does not promote greater weight loss in subjects who were prescribed an 8-week equi-energetic energy restricted diet'. *British Journal of Nutrition*, 2010 Apr;103(8)

[9] Hollis, J. 2008. "Weight Loss During the Intensive Intervention Phase of the Weight-Loss Maintenance Trial" *American Journal of Preventive Medicine*, 2008 Aug; 35(2): 118-126. doi: 10.1016/j.amepre.2008.04.013

[10] "Think before you eat: photographic food diaries as intervention tools to change dietary decision making and attitudes" *International Journal of Consumer Studies*, 2008, 32(6):692–698]

[8] *Which?* Rawstorne, T, 2015. "Are your ready prepared fruit & veg as healthy as you think? Tests show far lower levels of vitamin C than unprepared produce'

[9] Research by Martinez-Gonzalez, M, from University of Navarra, Spain. Smith, R, 2014, "Eating high fat yogurt lowers risk of obesity", *The Telegraph,* 31 May 2014.

[10] Lovallo, W R, et al, 2005. "Caffeine Stimulation of Cortisol Secretion Across the Waking Hours in Relation to Caffeine Intake Levels", *Psychosomatic Medicine.* 2005; 67(5): 734–739

CHAPTER 5

[1] Bajaj Wadhera, D, 2013. "Effect of Number of Food Pieces on Food Selection and Consumption in Animals and Humans", Arizona State University, May 2013.

[2] Golomb, B, et al, 2012. "Association Between More Frequent Chocolate Consumption and Lower Body Mass Index", *JAMA Internal Medicine, Arch Intern Med.* 2012;172(6):519–521.

[3] Flood, J E, Rolls, B J, 2007. "Soup preloads in a variety of forms reduce meal energy intake", *Appetite*, 2007 Nov; 49(3): 626–634

[4] Mosley, M, 2014. "Is reheated pasta less fattening?" BBC.co.uk; experiment conducted by van Tulleken, C, 2014, for *Trust Me I'm a Doctor* (BBC2, 2014)

CHAPTER 6

[1] Bezerra, I N, Sichieri R, 2009. "Eating out of home and obesity: a Brazilian nationwide survey" *Public Health Nutrition*, 2009 Nov;12(11):2037–43.

[2] Knäuper, B, et al, 2011. "Replacing craving imagery with alternative pleasant imagery reduces craving intensity", Appetite. 2011 Aug;57(1)

[3] Janssens P L H R, et al, 2013. "Acute Effects of Capsaicin on Energy Expenditure and Fat Oxidation in Negative Energy Balance", *PLOS One,* July 2, 2013

[4] Tharcilla Isabella Rodrigues Costa Alvarenga, et al, 2015. "Manipulation of Omega-3 PUFAs in Lamb: Phenotypic and Genotypic Views", *Comprehensive Reviews in Food Science and Food Safety*, Volume 14, Issue 3, pages 189–204, May 2015

[5] "Getting your omega-3s vs. a voiding those PCBs" *Harvard Health Publications, Harvard Medical School*, April 2004.

[6] Chan DS et al. Red and processed meat and colorectal cancer incidence: meta-analysis of prospective studies. PLoS One. 2011;6(6):e20456. Larsson SC, Wolk A. Red and processed meat consumption and risk of pancreatic cancer: meta-analysis of prospective studies. Br J Cancer. 2012 Jan 31; 106(3):603–7.

[7] Kirpitch, A R, Maryniuk, M D, 2011. "The 3 R's of Glycemic Index: Recommendations, Research, and the Real World" *Clinical Diabetes* October 2011 vol. 29 no. 4 155–159

[8] Jurenka, J S. 2009. "Anti-inflammatory properties of curcumin, a major constituent of Curcuma longa: a review of preclinical and clinical research", *Alternative Medicine Review*, 2009 Jun;14(2):141–53.

[9] Di Noia J. "Defining Powerhouse Fruits and Vegetables: A Nutrient Density Approach'. *Preventing Chronic Disease* 2014;11:130390

[10] Wansink, B, 2014. "*Slim By Design*", William Morrow

[11] Mohammed Saleem, T S and Darbar Basha, S, 2010. "Red wine: A drink to your heart" *Journal of Cardiovascular Disease Research*, 2010 Oct-Dec; 1(4): 171–176.

[12] Lippi G, et al. 2010. "Moderate red wine consumption and cardiovascular disease risk: beyond the "French paradox"", *Seminars in Thrombosis and Hemostasis*, 2010 Feb;36(1):59–70

[13] Galeaz, K, 2007. "*4 Weeks to Maximum Immunity: Disease-Proof Your Body*", Rodale. Research from Oregon State University, USA.

[14] Oh, H, Taylor, A H, 2013. "A brisk walk, compared with being sedentary, reduces attentional bias and chocolate cravings among regular chocolate eaters with different body mass", *Appetite*, 2013 Dec;71:144–9

[15] Bodenlos J S, Wormuth B M, 2013. "Watching a food-related television show and caloric intake. A laboratory study", *Appetite*, Volume 61, 1 February 2013

[16] University of Toronto, Canada, published in Journal of the Academy of Nutrition and Dietetics.

[17] Wansink B, van Ittersum K, 2012. "Fast food restaurant lighting and music can reduce calorie intake and increase satisfaction", *Psychological Reports*, 2012 Aug;111(1):228–32.

CHAPTER 7

[1] Yanovski S, 2003. "Sugar and Fat: Cravings and Aversions", *Journal of Nutrition*, March 1, 2003 vol. 133 no. 3

[2] Higgs S, 2008. "Recall of recent lunch and its effect on subsequent snack intake", *Physiology & Behaviour*, 2008 Jun 9;94(3): 454–62.

[3] Oh, H, Taylor, A H, 2013. "A brisk walk, compared with being sedentary, reduces attentional bias and chocolate cravings among regular chocolate eaters with different body mass", *Appetite*, 2013 Dec;71:144–9.

[4] Anshel M, 2014. "Applied Health Fitness Psychology", 2014, Human Kinetics. Research from the University of Texas Counseling and Mental Health Center

[5] Vohs K D, 2013. "Rituals Enhance Consumption", *Psychological Science*, Published online before print July 17, 2013

[6] McGonigal K, Steakley L, 2011. "The Science of Willpower", *Scope* (Stanford Medicine).

[7] Cunnane S C, et al, 2012. "Plasma and brain fatty acid profiles in mild cognitive impairment and Alzheimer's disease", *Journal of Alzheimer's Disease*, 2012;29(3):691–7.

[8] McGonigal K, Steakley L, 2011. "The Science of Willpower", *Scope* (Stanford Medicine).

[9] Koenders P G, van Strien T, 2011. "Emotional eating, rather than lifestyle behavior, drives weight gain in a prospective study in 1562 employees", *Journal of Occupational and Environmental Medicine*, 2011 Nov;53(11):1287–93.

[10] Peter P C, Brinberg D, 2012. "Learning Emotional Intelligence:

An Exploratory Study in the Domain of Health", *The Journal of Applied Social Psychology*, Vol 42, iss 6, June 2012

[11] Stuckey, H L , et al, 2011. "Using Positive Deviance for Determining Successful Weight-Control Practices", *Qualitative Health Research*, 2011 Apr; 21(4): 563–579

[12] Chang C Y, et al, 2009. "Essential fatty acids and human brain", *Acta Neurological Taiwanica*, 2009 Dec;18(4):231–41.

[13] Alcock J, et al, 2014. "Is eating behavior manipulated by the gastrointestinal microbiota? Evolutionary pressures and potential mechanisms", *Bioessays,* 2014 Oct;36(10):940–9.

[14] Bruinsma K, Taren D L, 1999. "Chocolate: food or drug?", *Journal of the American Dietetic Association,* 1999 Oct;99(10):1249–56.

[15] Wansink B, Payne CR, 2007. "Counting bones: environmental cues that decrease food intake'. *Perceptual and Motor Skills*, 2007 2007 Feb;104(1):273–6.

[16] Chao Y H, et al, 2012. "Food as ego-protective remedy for people experiencing shame. Experimental evidence for a new perspective on weight-related shame", *Appetite*, 2012 Oct;59(2):570–5.

[17] Wansink, B, 2014. "*Slim By Design*", William Morrow

[18] Zepeda L, Deal D "Think before you eat: photographic food diaries as intervention tools to change dietary decision making and attitudes" *International Journal of Consumer Studies*, [2008, 32(6):692–698]

[19] Dweck C S, Blackwell L S. "What is the Growth Mindset?"

[20] Pucciarelli, D L, 2013, "Cocoa and Heart Health: A Historical Review of the Science", *Nutrients*, 2013 Oct; 5(10)

[21] "Popcorn: The snack with even higher antioxidants levels than fruits and vegetables" Research by Dr J Vinson from the University of Scranton, US, presented at a meeting of the American Chemical Society.

[22] Cope E C, Levenson C W, 2010. "Role of zinc in the development and treatment of mood disorders", Current Opinion in Clinical Nutrition and Metabolic Care, 2010 Nov;13(6):685–9.

CHAPTER 8

[1] Tuttle B, 2011. "Study: Why You Should Shop for Groceries with a Cart, Not a Basket", *TIME*, July 20, 2011. Study originally published in *Journal of Marketing Research*, 2011.

[2 & 3] Maria L. Loureiro, Steven T. Yen, Rodolfo M. Nayga Jr. The effects of nutritional labels on obesity. *Agricultural Economics*, 2012; 43 (3)

[4] Fagherazzi G, et al, 2013. "Consumption of artificially and sugar-sweetened beverages and incident type 2 diabetes in the Etude Epidemiologique aupres des femmes de la Mutuelle Generale de l'Education Nationale-European Prospective Investigation into Cancer and Nutrition cohort", *American Journal of Clinical Nutrition*. 2013;97(3):517–23.

[5] Park K Y, et al. "Health benefits of kimchi (Korean fermented vegetables) as a probiotic food", *Journal of Medicinal Food,* 2014 Jan;17(1):6–20.

CHAPTER 9

[1] Laska M N, et al, 2014. "How we eat what we eat: identifying meal routines and practices most strongly associated with healthy and unhealthy dietary factors among young adults", *Public Health Nutrition,* 2014 Dec 2:1–11.

[2] Gorin A, et al, 2008. "Weight loss treatment influences untreated spouses and the home environment: evidence of a ripple effect", *International Journal of Obesity*, 2008 Nov;32(11):1678–84.

[3] Bright colors stimulate your appetite as well as your eyes Wansink, B, 2014. "*Slim By Design*", William Morrow

[4] Westerterp-Plantenga M S, et al, 2002. "Energy metabolism in women during short exposure to the thermoneutral zone", Physiology & Behaviour, 2002, 2002 Feb 1–15;75

[5] Stephens, Pippa, 2014. "Binge drinking link to overeating", bbc.co.uk, 24 April 2014.

[6] Prayson B, et al; 2008. "Fast food hamburgers: what are we really eating?", *Annals of Diagnostic Pathology*, 2008 Dec;12(6):406–9.

[7] Walker, Doug, Laura Smarandescu, and Brian Wansink (2013). "Half full or empty: cues that lead wine drinkers to unintentionally overpour", *Substance Use & Misuse*, 49(3), 295–302.

[8] Knapton, Sarah, 2014. "Secret to the perfect drink: serve it in a heavy glass, say experts", *The Telegraph*, 6 June 2014. Research from Professor Charles Spence, Oxford University.

[9] Gorelik S, 2008. "The stomach as a "bioreactor": when red meat meets red wine", *Journal of Agriculture and Food Chemistry*, 2008 Jul 9;56(13):5002–7.

[10] Marczinksi C A, Fillmore M T, 2014. "Energy drinks mixed with alcohol: what are the risks?", *Nutrition Reviews*, 2014 Oct;72 Suppl 1:98–107.

[11] Roberts C, Robinson S P, 2007. "Alcohol concentration and carbonation of drinks: the effect on blood alcohol levels", *Journal of Forensic and Legal Medicine*, 2007 Oct;14(7):398–405.

[12] Spence, C, 2014. "Noise and its impact on the perception of food and drink", *Flavor*, V3: 9

[13] Vidavalur R, et al; 2006. "Significance of wine and resveratrol in cardiovascular disease: French paradox revisited", *Experimental & Clinical Cardiology*, 2006 Fall; 11(3): 217–225.

[14] Rohsenow D J, et al, 2010. "Intoxication with bourbon versus vodka: effects on hangover, sleep, and next-day neurocognitive performance in young adults", *Alcoholism: Clinical and Experimental Research*, 2010 Mar 1;34(3):509–18.

[15] Insley, Jill, 2010. "Barbecue meals under fire for exceeding healthy calorie intake", *The Guardian*, 9 August 2010

[16] Martin F P, et al, 2009. "Metabolic effects of dark chocolate consumption on energy, gut microbiota, and stress-related metabolism in free-living subjects", *The Journal of Proteome Research*, 2009 Dec;8(12):5568–79.

[17] Wansink B, Kim J, 2005. "Bad popcorn in big buckets: portion size can influence intake as much as taste", *Journal of Nutrition, Education and Behaviour*, 2005 Sep-Oct;37(5):242–5.

CHAPTER 10
[1] Craft, L L; Perna, F M; 2004. "The Benefits of Exercise for the Clinically Depressed", *The Primary Care Companion—Journal of Clinical Psychiatry*, 2004; 6(3): 104–111.

[2] Burton JP et al (2012). Supervisor workplace stress and abusive supervision: the buffering effect of exercise. *Journal of Business and Psychology.*

[3] Karageorghis C I, et al, 2009. "Psychophysical and ergogenic effects of synchronous music during treadmill walking", *Journal of Sport & Exercise Psychology*, 2009 Feb;31(1):18–36.

[4] Ranganathan V K, et al, 2004. "From mental power to muscle power--gaining strength by using the mind", *Neuropsychologica*, 2004;42(7)

CHAPTER 11
[1] "Feeling powerless increases the weight of the world... literally", *University of Cambridge Research*, 4 February 2014. Report of research by Lee, E H, published in the *Journal of Experimental Psychology*, Feb 2014

[2] Cooper, Charlie, 2014. "Heart disease warning: Lack of exercise is worse risk for over-30s women than smoking or obesity", *The Independent*, 9 May 2014. Source: University of Queensland, Australia, *British Journal of Sports Medicine*, 2014.

[3] Westcott, W L, 2012. "Resistance training is medicine: effects of strength training on health", *Current Sports Medicine Reports*, 2012 Jul-Aug;11(4):209–16.

[4] Reynolds, G, 2014. "Younger Skin Through Exercise", *New York Times* (blogs, Well), 16 April 2014.

[5] Brito LB, et al, 2014. "Ability to sit and rise from the floor as a predictor of all-cause mortality", *European Journal of Preventive Cardiology*, 2014 Jul;21(7)

[6] Park, Alice, 2008. "Can exercise trump genetics?" *TIME*, 8 September 2008. Clinical study originally published in *Archives of Internal Medicine*, 2008.

[7] Oh, H, Taylor, A H, 2013. "A brisk walk, compared with being sedentary, reduces attentional bias and chocolate cravings among regular chocolate eaters with different body mass", *Appetite*, 2013 Dec;71:144–9.

[8] Kumanyika S K, et al; 2009; "Trial of family and friend support for weight loss in African American adults'. *Archives of Internal Medicine* 169(19) Oct 2009.

[9] Lee, D, et al; 2014. "Leisure-Time Running Reduces All-Cause and Cardiovascular Mortality Risk", *Journal of the American College of Cardiology*, 2014;64(5):472–481.

CHAPTER 12
[1] Oh, H, Taylor, A H; 2014; "Self-regulating smoking and snacking through physical activity", *Health Psychology*, 2014 Apr;33(4)

[2] McGonigal K, Steakley L, 2011. "The Science of Willpower", *Scope* (Stanford Medicine).

CHAPTER 13
[1] "The real-world benefits of strengthening your core", *Healthbeat, Harvard Health Publications*

[2] Buchanan K E, Bardi A; 2010. "Acts of kindness and acts of novelty affect life satisfaction", *The Journal of Social Psychology,* 2010 May–Jun;150(3):235–7.

[3] McKean, R, "Can caffeine improve sports performance?", *RunnersWorld. co.uk*

[4] Sim, A Y, et al, 2014. "High-intensity intermittent exercise attenuates ad-libitum energy intake", *The International Journal of Obesity*, 2014 Mar;38(3):417–22.

CHAPTER 14
[1] "Life At Home" report by IKEA, 2014 survey of over 2,000 people

[2] Blake K, 2012. "Anxiety relief lasts long after workout", *Futurity* (University

of Maryland, US), 20 Sep 2012. Originally reported in the journal *Medicine and Science in Sports and Exercise*.

[3] "Meditation improves the immune system, research shows", *The Telegraph*, 1 Nov 2011. Report from study published in the journal *Perspectives on Psychological Science*, Nov 2011.

[4] Kiecolt-Glaser J K et al, 2014. "Daily Stressors, Past Depression, and Metabolic Responses to High-Fat Meals: A Novel Path to Obesity", *Biological Psychiatry*, April 1 2015, Volume 77

[5] Stults-Kolehmainen M A, Bartholemew J B, 2012. "Psychological stress impairs short-term muscular recovery from resistance exercise", *Medicine & Science in Sports & Exercise*, 2012 Nov;44(11):2220–7.

CHAPTER 15
[1] Cohen, S, et al, 2012; "Chronic stress, glucocorticoid receptor resistance, inflammation, and disease risk", *Proceedings of the National Academy of Sciences of the United States of America*, 2012 Apr 17; 109(16): 5995–5999.

[2] Ahola, K, et al, 2012; "Work-Related Exhaustion and Telomere Length: A Population-Based Study", *PLOS One*, July 11, 2012

[3] Firger, J, 2014. "OMG, you're texting your way to back pain", *CBS News*, 14 November 2014

[4] "Exercise at work boosts productivity, Swedish researchers find", *ScienceDaily. com*, 8 September 2011.

[5] *The International Journal of Obesity*

[6] Adan A, 2012; "Cognitive performance and dehydration", *Journal of the American College of Nutrition*, 2012 Apr;31(2):71–8.

[7] Kosner, A, 2014. "Why The Best Time To Drink Coffee Is Not First Thing In The Morning", *Forbes*, 1 May 2014.

[8] Robinson A, et al, 2013. "Eating attentively: a systematic review and meta-analysis of the effect of food intake memory and awareness on eating", *The American Journal of Clinical Nutrition*, April 2013 vol. 97

CHAPTER 16

[1] Anwar Y, 2013. "Sleep deprivation linked to junk food cravings", *UC Berkeley News Center*, 6 August 2013

[2] "How to get to sleep", *NHS Choices*, 14 July 2014.

[3] "Consistent sleep patterns tied to healthier weight", *Medical News Today*, 19 Nov 2013.

[4] Jones C, Dawson D, 2012. "Eye masks and earplugs improve patient's perception of sleep", *Nurses Critical Care*, 2012 Sep-Oct;17(5):247-54.

[5] Mori Y, et al, 2002. "Effects of pressure on the skin exerted by clothing on responses of urinary catecholamines and cortisol, heart rate and nocturnal urinary melatonin in humans", *International Journal of Biometerology*, 2002 Dec;47(1):1-5.

[6] "Blue light has a dark side", *Harvard Health Publications*, 1 May 2012.

[7] Seppälä E M, et al, 2014. "Breathing-based meditation decreases posttraumatic stress disorder symptoms in U.S. military veterans: a randomized controlled longitudinal study", *Journal of Traumatic Stress*, 2014 Aug;27(4): 397-405.

[8] "Overcoming insomnia", *Harvard Health Publications*, 1 February 2011.

[9] Tasali, E, et al, 2014. "The effects of extended bedtimes on sleep duration and food desire in overweight young adults: A home-based intervention", *Appetite*, Volume 80, 1 September 2014, Pages 220–224.

WELCOME TO YOUR 12-WEEK FEELGOOD PLAN

[1] "Scientific Report of the 2015 Dietary Guidelines Advisory Committee. Part D. Chapter 5: Food Sustainability and Safety—Continued", *health.gov*

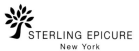

STERLING EPICURE
New York

An Imprint of Sterling Publishing
1166 Avenue of the Americas
New York, NY 10036

STERLING EPICURE is a trademark of Sterling Publishing Co., Inc. The distinctive Sterling logo is a registered trademark of Sterling Publishing Co., Inc.

This Sterling Epicure edition published in 2016

First Published in the UK in 2016 by Ebury Press, part of Penguin Random House UK

Text © 2016 by Dalton Wong and Kate Faithfull-Williams
Photography © 2016 by Philip North-Combes

ISBN 978-1-4549-1972-8

Distributed in Canada by Sterling Publishing c/o Canadian Manda Group, 664 Annette Street Toronto, Ontario, Canada M6S 2C8

For information about custom editions, special sales, and premium and corporate purchases, please contact Sterling Special Sales at 800-805-5489 or specialsales@sterlingpublishing.com.

Manufactured in Canada

2 4 6 8 10 9 7 5 3 1

www.sterlingpublishing.com

INDEX

THANK YOU

Dalton

"None of this would be possible without the support of my wife Christine, who has been absolutely central to my career, as well as being the best mother to Indigo and Ethan. Thank you Mom for raising me and Corrina; it must have been difficult at times, but I'm sure Dad would be proud of all of us.

"Thank you to my clients for shaping my philosophy about training and health. Special thanks goes to Jen (Team JL) for opening my eyes and so many doors, and thank you Nick for your continued support. Thank you Nigel for reminding me who the trainer is in our relationship; thank you Kit for being the most disciplined client (when asked nicely), and thank you Amanda for being so motivated.

"To Andrew White, thank you for all your advice in building TwentyTwoTraining into what it is today. Huge thanks to the best team: Dylan, George, Becky, Jane, Josh, David and Lucinda. Thank you to my mentors who have taught me to keep learning and to be an example to clients; that's you, Joe Gomes and Pat McGrath.

"Thank you Heather Dickinson for your social media support, thank you Sukeena Rao for your style advice, and thank you George Northwood for the best haircut in London.

"Huge thanks to all my training partners at Roger Gracie Academy who keep me humble and also in fantastic shape for an old man!

"My final appreciation is to Kate—without your drive and persistence this book would never have happened. Thank you. I'm very proud of our hard work and especially our message to enjoy life and food."

Kate

"Firstly, to my husband John-Rhys and our daughter Indy, my favorite people ever. Without you, neither this book nor my own personal feelgood plan would have been possible. Special thanks to my parents Jenny and Hugh Faithfull for adopting this book so enthusiastically, and to Alan and Beryl Williams, too.

"To my friends who shared their bright ideas: Jo Carnegie, Suzy Cox, Caroline Crowther, Laura Faithfull, Catherine Gray, Liz Hambleton, Leah Hearle, Erin Malone and Caroline Szumilewicz.

"To my gymspirational trainers, Josh Betteridge and David 'Baz' Hastie—you surprised me with my own strength and made me look forward to every sweat session.

"And finally, Dalton. Thank you for listening and saying yes, let's do this. It's been more fun than I ever could have imagined."

Thank you from both of us

"Thank you to our fantastic publishing team for literally putting our plan onto paper, especially our wise editor Lizzy Gray, genius designers Emma and Alex Smith, patient copy-editor Kay Halsey, behind-the-scenes magician Charlotte Portman, superstar publicists Claire Norrish, Sarah Bennie and Philly Vass, and our agent, Amanda Preston.

"Thank you to our shoot team: Alex Smith, Philip North Coombes, Jay Fenwick and Susie Kennett, who made Mallorca so much fun it felt like a holiday, just with really early starts. Sorry about that taxi bill. Thank you also to Anjhe Mules at Lucas Hugh, Deborah Hughes at Nike, and Ashleigh Stirling at Lululemon for your style expertise."